QUENCH

QUENCH

BEAT FATIGUE, DROP WEIGHT, AND
HEAL YOUR BODY THROUGH THE NEW
SCIENCE OF OPTIMUM HYDRATION

DANA COHEN, MD

GINA BRIA

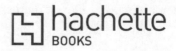

hachette
BOOKS

NEW YORK   BOSTON

Copyright © 2018 by Dana Cohen M.D. and Gina Bria
Illustrations by Alma Vescovi

Cover design by Amanda Kain
Cover copyright © 2018 by Hachette Book Group, Inc.

The Allergy Elimination Diet, excerpted from *Nutritional Medicine* by Dr. Alan Gaby, M.D. (Fritz Perlberg; 2011) in the Appendix, is reprinted with permission.

Hachette Books
Hachette Book Group
1290 Avenue of the Americas
New York, NY 10104
hachettebooks.com
twitter.com/hachettebooks

First edition: June 2018

Hachette Books is a division of Hachette Book Group, Inc.

The Hachette Books name and logo are trademarks of Hachette Book Group, Inc.

The publisher is not responsible for websites (or their content) that are not owned by the publisher.

The Hachette Speakers Bureau provides a wide range of authors for speaking events. To find out more, go to www.hachettespeakersbureau.com or call (866) 376-6591.

Library of Congress Cataloging-in-Publication Data

Names: Cohen, Dana, author. | Bria, Gina, author.
Title: Quench : beat fatigue, drop weight, and heal your body through the new science of optimum hydration / Dana Cohen, MD and Gina Bria.
Description: New York : Hachette Books, [2018] | Includes bibliographical references and index.
Identifiers: LCCN 2017055249| ISBN 9780316515665 (hardback) | ISBN 9781549168826 (audio download) | ISBN 9781549115370 (audio book) | ISBN 9780316515672 (ebook)
Subjects: LCSH: Nutrition. | Hydration. | Food habits. | BISAC: HEALTH & FITNESS / Healthy Living. | HEALTH & FITNESS / Nutrition. | HEALTH & FITNESS / Diets.
Classification: LCC RA784 .C5656 2018 | DDC 613.2—dc23
LC record available at https://lccn.loc.gov/2017055249

Printed in the United States of America

LSC-C

10 9 8 7 6 5 4 3 2 1

For our moms,

Bunny bunbuns,

and

Stephanie

Contents

Preface

Mni Wiconi.

—Lakota for "Water is life"

This book about hydration was inspired by two different authors from very different traditions: anthropologist Gina Bria and physician Dana Cohen. Each brought her own expertise and experience to this vitally important topic.

Gina was researching indigenous tribes from desert regions around the world and trying to understand how they survived drought conditions. At the same time, she was struggling to care for her elderly mother, who was in a nursing home seven hundred miles away. Gina eventually recognized that her mother was suffering from chronic dehydration, a health issue common to many residents of nursing homes. Like so many of us, her mom was subject to the dehydrating effects of indoor living in a sealed environment: artificial lighting, long hours of immobility, processed foods, medications, with little fresh air and sunlight, conditions almost drought-like in their drying effects.

Gina needed to figure out how to get her mom the hydration she so desperately needed. And in fact, that answer came from the very desert dwellers she was researching. They were experts in hydration. Instead of searching for water in their arid environment, they found their water another way. They practiced what so many of us today have forgotten—they used the water *locked in plants* to hydrate. Gina started focusing on the water already inside fresh food, such as apples, to help her mom get the hydration she needed, and the results were dramatic. Her mom never had another dehydration incident. Gina was amazed that no one was talking about this simple yet radically effective approach to wellness, and she started sharing her story about the power of water—particularly efficient plant water—in overall health.

Half a world away from these desert tribes, on the island of Manhattan, Dr. Dana Cohen was busy at her Midtown medical practice. Dr. Cohen is an integrative physician, one of a small but growing circle of New York City doctors moving away from prescribing medication for every ailment. Her holistic approach was tethered to the latest science in nutrition, which she offered her patients as an innovative way to promote health. She was always looking for new methods to help her patients, and she'd even been approached to write a book on the topic. She didn't want to write yet another generic health or diet title that focused on one area of wellness or one small segment of her patient population. She was looking for a far more universal message to accelerate healing for *all* her patients. And she was starting to experiment with a new protocol on some of them—treating them with not just nutrition, but also hydration. Her results showed early promise, and she wanted to amplify them.

One day, Gina and Dana found themselves in the same small office after several professional acquaintances had insisted that they meet. They soon realized that they had both been observing the same clues. Indeed, almost no one came into Dana's office without talking about their inexplicable fatigue and low energy. Could dehydration be behind so many pervasive complaints? Could better hydration be the upstream solution, intercepting decline? Gina talked passionately about her research. Desert dwellers were brilliant at harnessing plants to keep themselves hydrated for a much longer amount of time compared to city dwellers. It wasn't volume they were exploiting but absorption and retention. They ingested plants that *were already well hydrated.* She related her own personal experience seeing the dramatic effect that absorbed hydration had on her mother. Dana knew immediately that Gina was on to something.

"Think cactus," Gina told Dana, and she went on to tell her how she solved her mother's dehydration. "I got her to drink her orange juice, with chia seeds mixed in, to increase moisture retention by twofold."

Dana, too, had her own personal experience: Her mom had faded away in a nursing home fifteen years earlier from Alzheimer's, leaving Dana frustrated and hurt that as a young doctor she couldn't help her own mother. She also saw her patients coming into her office every day—frazzled, fatigued, unwell—and she had witnessed firsthand how returning them to a proper level of hydration could heal them. She just hadn't thought about using food as a tool for hydration until now.

Their conversation moved to the groundbreaking book written in 1992: *Your Body's Many Cries for Water,* by Fereydoon Batmanghelidj. Dr. Batman, as he was affectionately called, showed from his own clinical experience that dehydration can lead to many chronic conditions. To both Dana and Gina, this aligned with their belief that hydration should be used more by the scientific community as a key barometer of our health and that persistent low-grade dehydration is a larger factor in many chronic illnesses than currently understood. Dr. Batman's book, though still a substantial book on treating health issues with hydration, is over twenty years old. In the meantime, groundbreaking new findings on water have appeared.

Dana, sipping the smoothie Gina brought her, looked right

at her new partner and stated, "Let's write the new book on hydration."

That meeting planted the seed of an idea, and it has blossomed in amazing ways. Today, Gina is the head of the Hydration Foundation, a nonprofit organization that promotes the healing power and the new science discussed in *Quench*. And Dana continues her medical practice, incorporating these ideas in her hands-on work with hundreds of patients and sees dramatic results in the process.

The book you hold in your hands could be the answer to your own fatigue. Or headaches…brain fog…weight gain…insomnia…gut pain…joint pain. This book can elevate your smarts and cognitive performance at school and work, and protect you from sports injuries and concussion. We often mistakenly think these and other all-too-common modern maladies are due to gluten intake or too much sugar or too little exercise. But we identify a missing, and crucial, piece to the health puzzle that can no longer be overlooked. *Hydration* is our key to flourishing. In *Quench*, we give you entirely new and simple strategies based on breakthrough science and confirmed by ancient traditions. And we package it all in a five-day jump start plan, friendly and easy-to-do to get you to optimal hydration.

We have seen the dramatic, powerful health effects that come from understanding how optimal hydration can heal. And we're excited to share these healing techniques with you. Read on and start feeling better—today!

Hydration: How Can We Do It Better?

Water is life's matter and matrix, mother and medium. There is no life without water.

—*Nobel Prize winner Albert Szent-Györgyi*

For years, you've been told you need to drink eight glasses of water a day to get the hydration you need. And if you're trying to lose weight, you're feeling sick, or you're training for a big athletic event, eight glasses has always been just the tip of the (melted) iceberg. It's strange: In most aspects of our health, we are taught that moderation is the key. But the message when it comes to water has always been more, more, *more*. In our quest to be healthy, we've always thought we could never drink too much water.

The conventional wisdom was half right. Proper hydration *is* the key to unlocking optimal health. But we need to start looking at hydration for what it is: the very essence of your health. You are a body of water. In fact, by the most modest traditional estimates, approximately 65 percent of you is water. If you're not hydrated, everything else you do to stay healthy (exercising, eating right, stress management, sleep) is undercut.

It's known that humans can survive for about two months without food, but just days without water will kill us. Yet, shockingly, most of us are dehydrated—in fact, some doctors think as many as 75 percent of Americans are dehydrated.[1] Low-grade dehydration is the epidemic behind the epidemics, an omnipresent yet unseen dilemma tipped into new levels of urgency by our modern living conditions. What we eat—including salt-heavy, moisture-lacking processed food—makes our bodies work harder to metabolize. And a lack of hydrating greens and fruits keeps us dried out, even parched, all the time. In addition, we are ever more exposed to fluorescent lighting, dry heat, and air-conditioning…and that's not even considering all the electronic devices we use that further dehydrate us. On top of that, the very prescriptions and over-the-counter medications we take to reduce pain, stiffness, allergies, or any chronic condition are also very dehydrating. There is a long list of medications reported to the FDA that actually cause clinical dehydration. You may be using one right now. Think about the last time you took a Benadryl or Sudafed for allergies—surely, you felt these medicines' dehydrating effects. Are you taking aspirin or acetaminophen for a headache? Xanax or Ambien to help you sleep? Did anyone prescribe taking extra water with that?

Add in another surprising source of dehydration: immobility, which slows down or squelches water delivery into cells, as well as the all-important outflow of waste particles. All that sitting most of us do—usually in stale, artificial office air, or while riding in cars for hours—is literally dehydrating us by slowing our body's flow of water and energy.

As a result of all these factors, most of us live in a chronic level of dehydration. This shows up in us as fatigue, a lack of focus, and lowered mood, as well as poor sleep[2] and, surprisingly, even excess weight. In fact, according to a study by Dr. Tammy Chang and her colleagues[3] from the University of Michigan, people who are obese are more likely to be inadequately hydrated. And another study from the Department of Human Nutrition, Foods, and Exercise at Virginia Tech[4] showed that drinking water before a meal can improve weight loss. Brenda Davy, senior researcher on the study, states, "We found that over the course of twelve weeks, dieters who drank water before meals, three times per day, lost about five pounds more than dieters who did not increase their water intake."

The effects of chronic low-grade dehydration are real, long lasting, and potentially very debilitating. We believe this *hypo-hydration* is the mother of all epidemics and can be linked to many common ailments. The cues are afternoon fatigue, a decline in cognitive performance, headaches, weakness, urinary tract infections, and constipation. But some other disorders resulting from dehydration may come as a surprise: sleeplessness, decreased immunity, joint pain, chronic diseases like fibromyalgia, type 2 diabetes, reflux, and even Alzheimer's. We'll talk more about this in chapter 1, but suffice it to say that dehydration can have a big—and lasting—effect on our overall health.

So if we're hydrating all wrong, what are we supposed to do about it? That's where this book comes in. We know there's no one way to perfect health. But what if there was something that brought us closer? There's a *better* way to hydrate…and the benefits of proper hydration can have a dramatic effect on your health, your vitality, and your overall quality of life.

A BETTER WAY TO HYDRATE

Let us introduce you to a new way to claim the power of water. *Quench* will help you determine how to hydrate properly (hint: it doesn't involve chugging a gallon of water every day), and then how to get the water you do drink deep into your muscles, cells, and fascia (the connective tissue of your body), where it's needed most. When it comes to drinking enough water quantity is not necessarily quality. It's all about absorption, and that's why our plan will not push you to simply drink more. Why? Because counting on water alone to hydrate your body is inefficient— and it can even hurt you. Drinking too much water can flush out vital nutrients and electrolytes from your cells and tissues, actually harming your health and limiting your body's ability to perform. In chapter 2, we'll show why you need to incorporate more hydration into your diet not just through water but also through plants, such as fruits and vegetables, seeds, and other hydrating foods. The effects of hydration can be transformative, and once you feel them for yourself, you'll never look at a simple glass of H_2O the same way again.

So what *are* the benefits of proper hydration? For our kids, it can mean better mood and smarts. For athletes who want to perform better, stronger, and faster, proper hydration can be a game changer. For those of us who struggle with health issues like headaches, bloating, and even chronic diseases, getting the right kind of water can alleviate our symptoms and recharge our lives. And for our elders who struggle to get enough nourishment and hydration, this may actually be life-saving information. We can incorporate superhydrating foods into our diet in simple ways. We will help you find the best ways for you to hydrate deeply and completely—so that all your cells are quenched.

We have crafted a five-day jump start plan that offers you a delicious array of drinks, meal plans, and the heart of the program—smoothies—that all take advantage of the most hydrating and nutrient-packed foods to hydrate you more fully, more deeply, with longer retention. There is a *second* component to this plan that actually is the missing half of hydration. And that's moving water into your tissues. In chapter 3, we'll explain how movement delivers hydration. A key feature of this program is the inclusion of micromovements: small, simple movements you can do a few times a day that get the hydration into the tissues and organs that need it most. Chapter 4 outlines the science of micromovements. By doing our simple plan for five days, you will experience more energy, better focus, and improved digestion. We promise you will want to incorporate our hydration strategies and movements into a lifetime practice that will keep you moving without pain and living with a renewed vigor that you didn't know you had.

Are you dehydrated?

Take our self-assessment to determine if dehydration is affecting you:

Do you notice you can't seem to lose weight, even when trying?
Do you notice increased thirst?
Do you feel constipated?
Do you notice a decrease in your urine output?
Do you feel bloated?
Do you notice brain fog?
Do you have afternoon fatigue?
Do you struggle with daytime sleepiness?

Do you notice any dizziness?

Do you experience poor sleep?

Do you feel muscle stiffness?

Do you feel joint pain?

Do you have headaches?

Do you have dry skin?

Do you often have chapped lips?

Do you notice if your eyes are dry?

Do you notice if your mouth is dry?

Do you have bad breath?

Do you notice if your throat is dry?

Do you think you need to drink more water?

If you answered yes to any of these questions, your body may be signaling you that it needs hydrating. And consider it your first line of therapy. Tap water isn't enough.

Read on to find out how to get—and stay—hydrated. Your health depends on it.

OUR ENVIRONMENT IS DEHYDRATING

"But I drink plenty of water," you may be thinking. "How could I possibly be dehydrated?"

Even if we think we consume enough water, we are floating in low-grade fatigue, challenged by multiple moisture-stealing factors of today's way of life. If we think of a healthy body as if it were a plant—rooted in nutrient-rich soil, absorbing minerals and moisture, taking in sunlight and water and converting them into abundant greenery—then by contrast, today our hydration-deprived bodies are like wilted leaves and shriveled dry stalks. Do you sometimes feel that way?

It is estimated that humans lose two to three liters (about sixty to one hundred ounces) of water through breathing, sweat, urine, and bowel movements a day. Remember this adage: What goes in must come out, and vice versa. The delicate balance of water lost from the body must equal the amount of water taken in to maintain homeostasis (equilibrium) in our bodies.

If you're not fully replacing that water loss, your brain sends out hormone signals to divert water away from non-life-sustaining areas in order to regulate function of more important organs like your brain, heart, and liver. Thirst is not always an early-warning indicator of dehydration, so it is very easy to fall prey to low-grade dehydration without realizing it.[5] Dehydration can sneak up on you.

How do I know if I'm dehydrated?

Unfortunately, there's no exact science to determining whether you're chronically dehydrated; there's no reliable test your doctor can offer or a score by which you can measure your water level. But there are some good indicators that you may need more fluid in your body—try these self-tests at home to start to evaluate if your hydration can be improved.

- **Look at your urine.** As a general rule of thumb, urine color is a good "marker" of water intake. Urine is composed of water; urea (metabolic waste); organic materials, such as carbohydrates, enzymes, fatty acids, and hormones; and some electrolytes.

Normal urine should be clear to light yellow in color. It is often more yellow if you're taking vitamins or certain medications. Urine that is a dark yellow is an indicator of dehydration. Also watch for lower output.

- **Pinch your skin.** If it "tents"—it doesn't bounce back to its normal shape, especially on the tops of your hands—you are dehydrated.
- **Apply pressure to your fingernail for five seconds.** Release and observe the time it takes for the color to return to normal. Good hydration returns color in one to three seconds. If it takes longer than five seconds, you are likely dehydrated.
- **Keep track of your weight.** Weighing before and after exercise can be a little obsessive, but if you are exercising in a hot environment or you're doing a particularly long or strenuous activity, it can be prudent to monitor how much water you are losing. This is what elite athletes do—if you are endurance training and exercising for more than an hour at a time, make sure you are not losing too much water and, more important, that you are replenishing what you do lose. (See our recommendations in chapter 6.)

And think about the typical day in the office, where you barely get out the chair, perhaps even ordering in lunch. When you're immobile for long periods of time, your body struggles to deliver water into its cells and push out waste particles. All that sitting is literally dehydrating us by slowing our body's flow of water.

So should you start chugging twice as much H_2O as you already do now? Not so fast. New research reveals that you can hydrate better *and* smarter by taking a whole-health approach to hydration. And in doing so, you'll feel, function, and look your best. In *Quench*, we address everyday dehydration, not the advanced dehydration that could land you in the hospital with an IV drip. Instead we're here to show you how to replenish what you lose through daily functions: trips to the bathroom, perspiration, stress, and environmental hits like hot rooms, traffic jams, dry processed food, medications, and just modern living.

Even the smallest amount of dehydration can have a big impact: as little as a *2 percent* reduction in hydration leads to *measurable* cognitive loss.[6] That is less than one liter (or about thirty-three ounces) of water loss. Just enough for your sensory capacities to diminish. Apprehension diminishes and appreciation is depressed. Life is less colorful. That's your brain 2 percent dry. And *that* happens to most of us somewhere in our day. Often by three o'clock we are floating in low-grade dehydration, and by 9 p.m. we are sputtering near empty. Over and over, every day, through our lifetime, we dry out. This accelerates aging every day.

Dehydration can adversely affect almost every aspect of your health. Recent research from major universities, medical institutions, and even the U.S. Army reveal that even minor dehydration can make both major and minor aches—think joint pain, migraines, and postsurgical pain—worse.[7] It also thwarts your ability to focus[8] and *increases* your appetite.

But it doesn't have to be like this.

BOTTLED WATER ISN'T THE SOLUTION

You would think with all that we know about the importance of drinking water that we would be much better at keeping well hydrated. The truth is, we *should* be better hydrated than ever. After all, for most of us in the Western world, clean water is omnipresent—if not from our taps then in bottles. According to the Beverage Marketing Corporation, the sales of bottled water rose 7.9 percent in 2015, which is on top of a 7 percent increase in 2014. In 2016, Americans bought 12.8 *billion* gallons of bottled water. Bottled water is ubiquitous: Whether it's at a vending machine or on grocery store shelves, you can find water that comes from natural springs, water that's been purified by reverse osmosis, water with added electrolytes, and water mixed with coconut juice or aloe. Is there any science behind these additions and the claims that they're "good for you"? Are these expensive options really your only choices—and are they even the *best* choices—for healthy hydration?

Bottled water may be a healthy and increasingly common alternative to soft drinks, but the plastic bottle turns out to have a hidden dark side: energy consumption, waste disposal, and other environmental concerns. As bottled water grows in popularity, problems proliferate. Did you know...

- It takes three liters of water to produce a one-liter bottle of water.
- Worldwide, bottled water consumption more than doubled between 1997 and 2005, with U.S. residents tipping back the largest share—about 7.8 billion gallons total, or 26 gallons per person, in 2005.
- Bottled water costs as much as $10 per gallon compared to less than a penny per gallon for tap water.
- Fourteen percent of all litter comes from beverage containers.[9]

What a paradox that we drink so much water yet we can't keep pace with the dehydrating effects of modern life. Truth is, all this water has not eliminated dehydration—and bottled water isn't a viable short-term or long-term solution. Water shortages, record-setting droughts, and growing concerns over water pollution are ever-present reminders that we cannot take water, the fundamental element of life, for granted. We are urgently in need of a new approach to obtaining our everyday water. By habitually drinking bottled water, our society supports an industry that actually pollutes our environment and views water as a commodity rather than as a right and as indispensable to health for all living things. Bottled water is not only a less effective means of staying hydrated on the go, but it depletes aquifers and other sources of water, produces unnecessary waste, and is exorbitantly priced.

Alternatively, the Quench Plan for deep hydration, based on our understanding that *when* we drink is as important as what and how much, reshapes our attitudes surrounding this precious resource, while breaking our dependence on bottled water. Our method is sustainable and encourages readers to think more critically about the global impact of their drinking habits and fosters a healthier future for our water-challenged world.

WHAT DOES DEHYDRATION FEEL LIKE?

Along with problems around bottled water and beverages, misinformation abounds about what you should drink—as well as how and when. As mentioned earlier, thirst isn't always the most reliable warning of low hydration. Often when we feel fatigued or a headache coming on, we think we need to eat, but really we need to drink. Researchers speculate that these ill effects are your brain's built-in "alarm system," tipping you off to the fact that your body needs hydration ASAP. If you're feeling headachy, grumpy, unfocused, or otherwise less than great, chances are you're already dehydrated.

And the problems go beyond a fuzzy-headed feeling and a dry mouth. Research suggests dehydration is the link to many—if not most—ailments. As we'll discuss in more detail in chapter 1, dehydration contributes directly to a whole host of complaints, including:

- Headaches, including migraines
- Weakness and fatigue, both everyday and relating to conditions like fibromyalgia
- Foggy thinking and lack of focus
- Urinary tract infections
- Constipation
- Sleeplessness
- Decreased immunity
- Heart disease
- Type 2 diabetes
- Acid reflux
- Dementia, including Alzheimer's disease

HYDRATE SMARTER

How do desert cultures hydrate?

The Bedouins, Arabian desert nomads, know a thing or two about hydration. They gulp, not sip, their liquid. They give their organs a good soak first thing in the morning and then get on with the day's travel. That is one of their key strategies that results in the need for less liquid. Because adult Bedouins' daily water intake averaged only one liter, anthropologists had a hard time under-standing how they could survive under such harsh desert condi-tions. But they didn't account for the Bedouins' food intake. Camel or goat milk was the foundation of Bedouin hydration, as was a form of goat butter or ghee slathered on bread and used in cooked dishes. Both milk and butter provide high levels of electrolytes. Ethnographic anecdotes also reveal that Bedouins traveled under those heavy black robes to create a humidifying tent with their breath and perspiration, creating, in essence, a portable moisten-ing microenvironment.

We don't know enough about water, this most common element. Scientists and doctors are still mystified as to how the water mol-ecule actually functions, how it aids health, and exactly how much is really needed to stay hydrated. There is still no stan-dardized way to measure adequate hydration in our bodies. But what we are finding out is that hydration is more critical to our health than we know, and now more than ever.

Fortunately, new exciting research emerges every day. One very important finding is how water affects our over-all health by potentially intercepting chronic conditions. We've combed through the research for you and put together a com-prehensive picture of how to drink smarter. Protecting yourself from chronic conditions is not about increasing intake but about how well your body absorbs water. Groundbreaking studies—still being conducted in and beyond the science lab—show that water locked in plants hydrates more efficiently and fully than plain tap water alone. How? Plant fibers help us absorb all that liq-uid, which has revolutionized the way we think about hydration.

PLANT WATER HYDRATES BEST

Plants—leafy greens, fruits, vegetables, roots and seeds—have always been known for good nutrition. But we are now discovering that consuming the water contained in plants is better than drinking water alone. It is already purified, alkaline, pH perfect, mineralized, full of nutrients, structured (more about that later), and energized to absorb easily into our cells. Think about that the next time you eat a deliciously ripe peach. The juice that trickles down your chin is a different, more potent kind of water. We have early findings from researchers that show that this plant water is likely the most efficient way to hydrate. Smart Mother Nature, and great packaging!

Because these studies are so new, no adequate clinical work yet confirms how well plant water hydrates. But the Quench Plan springboards off this exciting research. Over the past two and a half years, we have been working with more than four hundred patients on improving their hydration status and have seen amazing results that improve their health and quality of life.

What you hold in your hands is a culmination of our research and case studies that make our Quench program so effective.

THE QUENCH PROGRAM

As an integrative physician and a cultural anthropologist, we have combined our research and years of practical experience with this new information. *Quench* will help you get more water into your body by blending vegetables and fruits and other ingredients with water, all designed for maximum hydration.

The plan's healthy mix of a plantcentric diet, including

smoothies, soups, and other hydrating meals, are complemented by our "recipes" of easy micromovements. These micromovements are designed to draw hydration deep into your cells. The movements can be seamlessly incorporated into your day, no matter where you are and no matter your level of physical fitness.

While the scientific community is still identifying how plants improve hydration in the cells, we have seen the results in those who have already used the Quench Plan. What we and others have seen is that by using plant water, we not only gain nutrition, we also benefit from better hydration through absorption.

You'll find your energy levels soar because you finally absorbed enough water. Most important, though, water will improve your body's functions in every way and fortify your body to help prevent weight gain, slow the aging process, and protect against disease. Don't take our word for it: In this book, we will include case studies from patients who have benefited from the Quench Plan and share how their lives have changed for the better. We will also provide fascinating insights from anthropological research that confirm that many ancient and indigenous peoples found an optimal way to best hydrate—with plants. The goal here is to bring together these ancient practices and align them with modern science and clinical results.

You will feel the effects of our five-day program right away and see concrete results over the weeks and months to follow. We've rooted our method in traditional techniques used in cultures all over the world—who have in their own way conducted clinical trial and error over eons of use—and we've only confirmed it with other scientists and health practitioners.

We use these methods ourselves, and we've helped hundreds of others feel and look better by following the right hydrating routine, one that your body can easily absorb. Our recommendations for hydration will not only quench your thirst, they will also infuse your body with vital nutrients. Now you can create a practical, healthful routine that will raise your hydration to levels you've never experienced before.

To get you on your way, here's our go-to Quench Plan rules that are based on the following three principles of hydration. We will lay out all the details for you in upcoming chapters:

1. **Drink for maximum absorption.** Get the maximum absorption from the water you drink, and make it available all the way down to the cellular level. How to do this?
   - When you first wake up, drink 8 to 16 ounces of water with a pinch of sea salt and the squeeze of a lemon to truly soak your insides.
   - Drink at least one green smoothie every day.
   - Drink 6 to 8 ounces of water before every meal.
   - Move.

2. **Get more of your water from food.** Eating foods high in water content can boost deep hydration—our plant-rich smoothies, for instance, will hydrate you far better than the *same amount of bottled water*. We'll show you how to incorporate more hydrating foods into your meals.

3. **Use movement to distribute hydration.** We'll show you easy-to-do yet crucial micromovements to deliver hydration more deeply into your tissues to keep you flexible and pain free.

DR. DANA'S CASE STUDY

Elizabeth

Elizabeth is a healthy fifty-six-year-old flight attendant. She's in generally good health, but flying has taken its toll on her body. As we all know, flying is extremely dehydrating: It results in dry skin, fatigue, brain fog, muscle aches—you name it, Elizabeth had it. At her age, she was concerned about menopause, even though she didn't have any major symptoms like hot flashes or vaginal dryness. Many sufferers would exclaim, "Lucky girl!" Elizabeth had read up on hormone replacement, and she thought it could help her alleviate her general "blah" feeling, as she called it. But when she came to see me, looking for a prescription for hormones, I suggested looking deeper together before putting her on hormone replacement therapy (HRT). While I freely prescribe bio-identical hormones, my philosophy is "less is more," and it wasn't clear Elizabeth needed hormone therapy—so we decided to run some tests first.

While we waited for the tests to come back, I put Elizabeth on the Quench program. When Elizabeth returned for a follow-up three weeks later, she couldn't believe the results. Fatigue, gone. Brain fog, cleared up. Aches, disappeared. I also noticed that Elizabeth's skin was glowing. "I can't believe it—I just feel my energy has bounced back—and I have noticed I am not as tired after a long flight. And I have more patience with difficult passengers!"

We talked about HRT: All of Elizabeth's initial blood work had come back normal, and she seemed to do so well with the Quench program, so it seemed that she didn't need hormone replacement therapy yet. She continued on the program—and she also shared it with her fellow flight attendants. At her next checkup several months later, Elizabeth told me that everyone who tried it also noticed a huge shift in their energy, skin, and mental clarity, and they had less aches and pains in general. They have all stuck to the plan—and they even joke with one another about their stashes of chia seeds on the plane to fold into their drinks while flying.

Why do I get so thirsty when I fly?

We can certainly count airplanes as one of the worst of modern dehydrating environments. Everybody knows it; everybody feels it. Dehydration, not jet lag, is the foremost reason why it is so exhausting to fly. In addition, the recirculated air on airplanes has less humidity than we are used to, dehydrating us further. Airplane cabins are often less than 20 percent humidity, unlike the 50 percent humidity in which we need to live comfortably. And long flights are even worse—a cross-country or transcontinental flight can have as little as 1 percent humidity. This drives our thirst, and our lips, eyes, and nose can dry out. Here are some great tips to keep in mind the next time you are jet-setting:

- **As a general guide, drink one 8-ounce glass of water for each hour of flying time.** Buffer it with a little natural salt. Don't flush out your minerals without any incoming electrolyte replacement. Carry a little packet or ziplock bag of natural salts, and pinch some in your water bottle. We prefer a bottle of water, salted naturally, and an apple over two bottles of water. The fiber in the apple will help you stay moist longer.
- **Carry a small bag of chia, pumpkin, hemp, or sunflower seeds.** An excellent strategy is to grind any of these seeds in your coffee grinder and toss and shake at least a tablespoon right in

your drink. Or you can snack on them as you are drinking. They will help absorb and add additional energy to the water you drink.

- **Plane posture is a real factor in keeping your flow going during flight.** Here's a trick for better posture on a plane: Sit up straight for a moment, then stuff a jacket, sweater, pillow, or even a book between your back and the plane seat. Place it so it lines up across from your belly button. This is the sweet spot that presses your whole spine into alignment and lengthens your spinal canal, putting all that synovial fluid into maximum flow. Now you will be able to work with laser-sharp focus.

- **Get up and go to the bathroom, even if you don't have to pee.** Movement and leg stretching at least every hour means you won't land tired. If your seat partner seems annoyed at having to move, just secretly rejoice that you are probably saving them, too, from further fatigue or even a deep vein thrombosis attack, since blood clots are a real risk after long periods of immobility. See chapter 1 for more details.

- **Do micromovements throughout the flight.** Chin to Chest, Ear Meets Shoulder, and use your shoulder blades to massage your seat back. See Quench plan micromovements, chapter 8.

- **Give yourself a facial.** You can gently massage your temples and behind your ears. You will just look like you have a headache, but you will be moving fluids into key spots to reduce fatigue.

- **Hydrate your face and hands.** Any cream with aloe vera is a super buffer against the dry and recirculated air on a plane. It acts as a barrier to keep what moisture you have in; not only is it hydrating, but it contains antibacterial and antiviral properties. You can further help yourself by applying lotion to your nasal area to keep your nasal passages hydrated, which allows you to better fight off airborne contaminates.[10]

You'll be amazed at the effects optimal hydration will have on your body:

- You'll have better concentration and will lose the brain fog that affects so many of us.
- Your energy will soar, overcoming fatigue that is often brought on from dehydration.
- You will experience improved digestion, elimination, and toxin removal as cellular function in every system in your body will be more effective.
- You will sleep better and deeper. No kidding. Let water do what no herbal remedy or prescription can do.
- Your flexibility will improve as your joints, muscles, and fascial system are adequately lubricated. Believe it or not, even our bones are about 31 percent water.
- You weight loss plan will finally work. Water is one of the best tools for weight management, so that yo-yo weight will be a thing of the past.
- You will eliminate bloating and swelling. No swollen ankles! Your clothes will fit better.
- Your skin will be radiant and younger looking—water "plumps" the skin with its moisture.
- Inflammation will diminish as our waste systems improve.

PLANTS AND THE EARTH

The discovery that plants hold a major role in hydration couldn't have come at a more critical time. Access to clean and sufficient water is a pressing social issue, and concern about water scarcity and purity is on the rise. Severe droughts are becoming more frequent, placing more pressure on global water supplies. *Quench* combines old strategies used all along by ancient traditions with new water science to hydrate *efficiently*. Simply put, by following our plan, you can ingest less water and still be better hydrated, nourished, and more flexible. This efficient approach to water consumption helps both our bodies and our planet. *Quench* offers a new approach that is a vitally important part of a natural and permanent solution and available to all.

Read on and experience for yourself what *quenching* your body can do for you.

CHAPTER 1

The New Science of Water

The Hydration/Health Connection

Nothing is softer or more flexible than water, yet nothing can resist it.

—*Lao Tzu*

Hydration is an essential human need, yet we foolishly continue to underestimate its importance. Your level of hydration impacts the strength of your immune system, the elasticity of your skin, your energy level, how easily you can move, and your body's overall resistance to aging and disease. It even determines how good you feel when you get up in the morning.

As science continues to gain a fuller understanding of how hydration works—and as we'll emphasize in this book, it doesn't just involve drinking eight glasses of water a day—how much you drink is only the first part of the story. We now know that what you drink, when you drink, and how your body moves liquid into its cells are crucial factors in achieving optimum health and feeling good. Let's take a closer look at the science of water and hydration.

THE ELUSIVE MEASUREMENT OF WATER

There are multiple ways to determine how much water we are made up of, and that isn't even taking stock of when and where it's measured. For example, babies are 75 percent water, while the elderly can be as low as 55 percent—we lose hydration as we get older. Inside us, water is moving around and changing form and function, becoming blood or vapor or joint fluid. To understand all those functions, we need a more sophisticated way of measuring water.

Brian Richter, a respected water research scientist, took a crack at the math. In a 2012 post on *National Geographic*'s website called "Walking Water," he postulates:

Imagine carrying 120 pounds of water... around with you all day long, every day of the year. No wonder I'm so tired at the end of the day... Add another 24 pounds of skin and what you've basically got is hundreds of thousands of years of human evolution producing an ambulatory water balloon wrapped in flesh... During a normal day, we breathe, pee, and sweat out about three quarts of water, amounting to 5–10 percent of our body's water.

With a loss of even a quart of water, Richter explains, you're likely going to start losing some cognitive function, alertness, and ability to concentrate. "If you lose a gallon ... you'll likely have a bad headache. If you're down two gallons you're going to be sick enough to be in the hospital. Three gallons and you're in the morgue."

To really understand how water works for us, let's look

at how it affects us at the molecular level. In this molecular world, you are made not of 60 percent water, or 70 percent water, or even 75 percent water, but 99 percent water. How can that be? If that were true, wouldn't that make us just a liquid puddle? To even get to that 99 percent number, we have to count all the molecules of matter in the body. When we do that, we find that 99 out of every 100 of them are water. This is because water is the tiniest of molecules. Needless to say, that is a lot of H_2O in our bodies. Let's examine what all that water is doing there.

WATER DOES THE BODY GOOD

How can one simple oxygen and two hydrogen atoms do so much?

Water molecules contain a polar arrangement between oxygen and hydrogen atoms—hydrogen has a positive electrical charge, while oxygen's is negative. This allows the molecule to attract many other types of molecules, such as salt (NaCl). Water can dissolve salt because the hydrogen attracts the negative chloride ions and negative oxygen attracts the positive sodium ions. Substances that dissolve easily like sugar and salt are hydrophilic, and those that don't—like oil—are called hydrophobic.

It isn't only water's *chemical* composition that makes it an excellent solvent—which means that wherever it travels, either through the ground or through our bodies, it takes along valuable chemicals, minerals, and nutrients into our cells. It is also H_2O's *molecular* configuration that lets water carry things into and out of our cells. In effect, water disassembles material at the molecular level.

And this simple yet complex molecule is *the* first line of defense for our body as it helps maintain homeostasis in our cells. Water helps keep this critical balance by performing five critical functions:

1. **Water promotes cell function.** Water is like an irrigation system; it helps bring nutrients (vitamins, minerals, carbohydrates) and oxygen in and out of every cell—without water, cells will die.
2. **Water helps maintain temperature regulation.** When our body temperature rises, we produce sweat that cools the body down.
3. **Water gets rid of our waste products** by urination and sweat, of course, but it also helps rid our bodies of solid waste.
4. **Water is a great lubricant.** It helps absorb shock; it acts like grease for our joints and tissues; it is a protectant to our organs; it cradles our brain in our cranium; it lubricates our eyes, nose, and mouth, making it easier to eat, breathe, and cry.
5. **Water is essential for our body's chemical and metabolic reactions.** Water participates in the biochemical breakdown of what we eat in the form of proteins, lipids, and carbohydrates. Basically, H_2O helps us break down everything we need from food into energy and helps us eliminate what we don't need.

YOUR BODY'S INNER IRRIGATION SYSTEM

Whether you drink water or eat water-rich foods, you know that liquid ends up in your stomach, where some of it is sent to your bloodstream to nourish your tissues and another percentage is sent through your digestive system.

As it happens, your bloodstream isn't the only way water reaches your organs and other areas of our body where it's needed. Exciting and important new research reveals that fascia—layers of spongy tissue found not only just under your skin but around your organs, muscles, nerves, blood vessels, and bones—doesn't just wrap and hold all your parts together. It's also an intricate water delivery system that sends water directly to the areas it's needed. We'll explore the importance of hydration and fascia in chapter 3, but know that every time you drink water, you're feeding your body's complex and beautiful fascial tissue.

HYDRATION AND DISEASE

On a more macro level, we know that water helps the body stave off a number of chronic diseases and conditions. So much so that we and many other experts would go as far as to say that water is quantitatively the most important nutrient to consider when looking at the origins of chronic issues. It definitively plays a role in a variety of health issues all of us will deal with as we age.

Cardiovascular Conditions, Including Coronary Heart Disease, Stroke, Hypertension, and High Blood Pressure

Would you believe that even mild dehydration—to the tune of just a 2 percent decrease in hydration levels—can impact your blood vessels the same way smoking a cigarette does? It's true. A new University of Arkansas study found that young men who don't hydrate optimally experience an immediate decrease in the ability of their endothelium's (that's the lining of their blood vessels) ability to constrict and dilate—functions that are essential for healthy blood flow.[1] If that's what happens to adults in ideal health, imagine the effects for those of us who are older or have heart disease risk factors like diabetes. No surprise, experts at Harvard say even low levels of dehydration ups your odds of suffering a heart attack.[2]

Why? It's actually pretty easy to visualize: When there's less water in your blood, it becomes thicker. As cardiologist Stephen Sinatra, MD, notes, healthy blood has the consistency of wine; it shouldn't be like a watered-down version of ketchup. But that's exactly how thick your blood can become, and quickly, if you're not adequately hydrated. Thick blood makes your heart work harder to pump, which can damage your heart muscle and contribute to high blood pressure. It also forces your body to use more energy to make blood flow through your arteries and capillaries—energy that could be better used in other areas of your body, like your brain. The result is a combination of cellular inflammation and heart and blood vessel issues that set the stage for cardiovascular disease. Dr. Sinatra's work in integrative cardiology has led him to expand his research on electrical impulses in the body beyond just the heart and how water affects this conduction. We will tell you more about the vital importance of water and electricity further on.

Diabetes

If you have type 1 or type 2 diabetes, you're already at a higher risk for becoming dehydrated. That's because your body's inability to make insulin (as with type 1 and advanced type 2 diabetes) or insensitivity to insulin (type 2) can lead to higher blood sugar levels, also known as hyperglycemia. Why is that an issue? When your blood sugar level is high, your kidneys will try to remove it from your bloodstream by creating extra urine. Over-urinating leads to—you guessed it—dehydration.

It's a cyclical problem: The thicker and less hydrated your blood is, the higher your blood sugar levels are likely to be, simply by virtue of the fact that there's not enough water to dilute all that sugar. As a result, you can get even more dehydrated, which leads to additional blood sugar problems.

The result can be a serious condition called ketoacidosis, which appears when your blood sugar levels are too high, your insulin levels are too low, and your body begins burning fat for energy, letting off high levels of potentially toxic blood acids called ketones in the process. You might have heard of ketones as a weight-loss strategy promoted by high protein diets, but for people with diabetes, those ketones can be deadly.[3]

What helps prevent this cycle? Adequate fluid intake, of course. By staying properly hydrated, you'll also lower your risk of heart disease and high blood pressure, which are higher than average for people with insulin-dependent diabetes.[4]

Some experts even think hydration can lower your risk of *developing* type 2 diabetes. When you're chronically dehydrated, the little water you do consume goes straight to the organ that's arguably most vital for helping you stay alive: your brain. Because of this, the water volume in your bloodstream diminishes, leading by a series of metabolic processes to higher blood sugar levels. If this happens every once in a while, it is unlikely to harm your health. But repeated day after day, week after week, dehydration causes chronic high blood sugar levels—which damage your body's sensitive cells. This makes them less responsive to the effects of insulin. That's insulin resistance, which can quickly turn into type 2 diabetes.[5]

Digestive Issues

Whether you're regularly constipated or crampy (or both), upping your water intake and filling your diet with water-rich foods can help turn your gut woes around. Perhaps the primary reason: Water and water-rich foods like chia and vegetables (which are also high in digestion-aiding fiber) help soften your food during digestion and soften your stool, too. And when your stool is soft, it passes through your system faster and more easily, preventing gut pain and bloating and improving your ability to eliminate waste without straining or resorting to laxatives. According to the health professionals at Barnard College, laxatives are themselves dehydrating and in turn compensate by retaining water and thereby causing more bloating.[6]

Water can help aid more serious digestive issues as well, like acid reflux or ulcers, as surmised by Dr. Batmanghelidj in his book *Your Body's Many Cries for Water*. Batmanghelidj had been a political prisoner in Iran in the late 1970s. During that time he treated and healed thousands of his fellow prisoners, many of whom had peptic ulcer disease, with nothing but water and electrolytes in the form of salt or sugar.[7]

The Hydrating Power of Chia

Chris McDougall's bestselling book, *Born to Run: A Hidden Tribe, Superathletes, and the Greatest Race the World Has Never Seen*, introduced thousands of readers to the Tarahumara tribe in the desert canyons of the Sierra Madres, whose young men run fifty-mile marathons for *fun*. In the book, McDougall described how the Tarahumara fuel themselves for the marathons with chia seeds. Before the run, they drink a mixture of fermented corn beer and chia seeds and took with them a small pouch filled with only about two tablespoons of additional chia seeds. Unbelievable: Here were a desert people showing enormous endurance by running a distance that seemingly exceeded what is humanly possible—without hydrating themselves with gallons of water but instead simply ingesting a tiny local seed. Each seed, we are finding out, enabled these long-distance runners to provide themselves with slow-release hydration as they ran. Those misleadingly dry-looking chia seeds hold an integral ingredient that the runners needed: When mixed with liquid, they release a form of gelled water that hydrates more slowly and effectively over time than liquid alone.

If you have a chronic digestive problem like Crohn's disease, colitis, or irritable bowel syndrome, adequate water intake is a must because each of these conditions cause diarrhea, which makes your body lose more water than it would otherwise.

Deep Vein Thrombosis, aka DVT

DVT can occur when a blood clot forms deep in your veins (typically in one of your legs). It most often affects travelers—though if you're pregnant, are using estrogen–based birth control, are overweight or obese, are elderly, have reduced circulation in your lower legs, or have recently had surgery, you're also at a higher risk.

DVT is a serious condition that can lead to a pulmonary embolism, which is a blockage of a blood vessel in your lung; it's often fatal. Hydration helps prevent DVT in two ways: one, by keeping your blood from thickening and forming clots; and two, by increasing your need to urinate, which makes you move more often. Even small bursts of physical activity lower your risk of DVT.

That's why it's so important to skip dehydrating alcoholic drinks and opt for water—and plenty of it—when you're flying or taking long car trips. The same is true if you have any of the DVT risk factors just mentioned.[8]

Pulmonary Disorders, Including Chronic Obstructive Pulmonary Disorder (COPD) and Asthma

Water keeps all your body's inner workings lubricated and functioning the way they should—and your airways and lungs are no exception. Water thins the mucus lining in your lungs and throat. Healthy mucus helps your body process and discard inhaled pollutants, toxins, and other substances that can pose a risk (both to healthy lungs and those affected by problems like COPD). Mucus that's thick and unhealthy filters fewer breathing-impairing substances—which explains why dehydration makes COPD (in the form of chronic bronchitis or emphysema) worse. Some research even suggests that dehydration may contribute to inflammation in the airways, which makes it harder to breathe.[9]

DR. DANA'S CASE STUDY

Hank

Hank is a thirty-year-old computer analyst. He has long struggled with his weight, which had fluctuated widely since his teens. In his early twenties the scales tipped at 250—at only five nine, he was obese. That was a turning point for Hank. Determined to lose the weight, he started a vigorous exercise regimen and a strict low-carb, high-protein diet. He lost seventy pounds within the year. At one point, he worried that he might be on the verge of becoming anorexic, as he whittled his weight down to 150. But after slipping back to bad eating habits, he ballooned back up to 240.

Beyond frustrated, he came to see me.

"Help me. I don't know why I have such an issue with my weight."

"Let's see what's going on." I reassured him.

After doing a round of routine blood tests and an exam, I went through his medications. Hank has had asthma for as long as he can remember, and he used an albuterol inhaler (a rescue inhaler) every day. He also took medication for anxiety. He smoked half a pack a day, exercised twice a week, mixing it up with both weights and cardio. His typical daily diet:

Breakfast—a small bagel with cream cheese, two cups black
   coffee
Lunch—salad with grilled chicken and feta cheese, drizzled with
   olive oil
Dinner—a Subway six-inch sandwich of turkey on a white roll

I was concerned that food sensitivities might be causing his weight fluctuations and possibly affecting his asthma, so I decided to put Hank on an elimination diet (see more about this in the pages that follow). I also suggested that he increase his hydration by drinking two glasses of water with lemon and sea salt in the morning, as well as a glass of water before every meal, and one to two additional glasses after every workout. I also gave him a recipe for a breakfast smoothie that included elimination-diet-friendly greens, pea protein, berries, coconut milk, and hydrating chia.

He returned three weeks later *nine* pounds lighter! He couldn't believe it, and I was pleasantly surprised, too. He told me he felt lighter and more energized, and more important, he felt *better*. He felt as if a huge weight had been lifted. We went over his lab results, which were all normal, except his environmental allergies—they were off the charts.

A year later, Hank is a much slimmer version of himself, at around 195 pounds. He is on different inhaler that he uses twice a day—a non-steroid medication called salmeterol—and he has not had to use his rescue inhaler at all. I put him on Singulair—an antiallergy medication that decreases lung inflammation with very few side effects. The best thing is that he has kicked the smoking habit, although he still uses nicotine gum. With his energy soaring, he works out religiously four times a week. He continues to hydrate efficiently, and he says he notices a difference if he skips his morning smoothie. He has slowly incorporated many foods back into his diet (except for shellfish—because he's very allergic), but he continues to avoid gluten and dairy. A real *Quench* success story!

NOTE: The elimination diet is a great place to start for anyone with any undiagnosed chronic ailment, as hidden food sensitivities can be a frequent cause of a wide range of medical issues.[10] In fact, I urge almost every patient who walks through my door to do an elimination diet. And I have seen life-altering results. Why? Food sensitivities are an underexplored cause of chronic illnesses, such as irritable bowel, migraines, asthma, allergies, and muscle and joint pain. And maybe even more important, these sensitivities often lead to *future* chronic disease. I believe if we avoid offending foods, we could be avoiding possible triggers for illness—like autoimmune diseases and possibly the big "C," cancer.

Food sensitivities are different from true food allergies like peanut allergies where your throat tickles—or worse, swells. Most adults already know if they have these acute allergic reactions to foods, but food sensitivities are not so easily uncovered or as easily tested for. That's where an elimination diet comes in.

We have included in the appendix a very comprehensive allergy elimination diet by Dr. Alan Gaby, but for a quick, down-and-dirty elimination diet, I have patients eliminate the five most common food sensitivities for twenty-one days: gluten, dairy, eggs, corn, and soy. After that three-week period, they reintroduce each food group, one at a time. I have them eat the food every day twice a day for three days and journal what happens to them. Symptoms can be anything from gas, bloat, diarrhea, constipation, or fatigue, to headache, skin rash, joint or muscle pain, or brain fog. If no symptoms occur after three days, the patient goes on to the next food, reintroducing it in the same way and tracking symptoms similarly. If symptoms occur, I tell them to eliminate the food and go on to the next food, and so on.

You may be asking, "All this sounds great, but why get into an elimination diet mentioned in a book about hydration?" As we have laid out, so much about hydration is about repairing our body after injury and protecting us from disease. Think of our Quench Plan and the elimination diet as a one-two punch. When used together, they powerfully provide protection from chronic illness. We include both of them in the book in hopes you do them together. And you can do this as long as you choose from the foods that are allowed on the diet. The two together are often a life-changing experience for patients.

We strongly recommend that before starting the elimination diet you consult with a trained health care professional who knows your health history, because if the regimen is not followed properly, it can lead to nutritional deficiencies. An elimination diet might not be recommended for people with severe asthma or severe eczema. Of course you can always start gently with just the five-day Quench Plan and still see amazing results.

Your Brain and Cognition

Yes, you want to improve your health. But what really motivates most of us to take action is a desire to *feel* better. And water can do that for you—in numerous ways. If you've noticed that you feel foggy or unfocused, water is an almost immediate fix. A 2012 study in the *Journal of Nutrition* found that even mild dehydration lowered women's concentration levels and they performed poorly on tests that measured cognition and focus.[11] Conversely, they were able to perform these tests well when they were fully hydrated. Dehydration also lowered women's moods. And women aren't the only ones affected by dehydration: Other research shows that drinking water improves memory and focus in children and men, too.[12]

Why do men have a higher percentage of water than women? Muscles are about 75 percent water, and men have a slightly higher percentage of muscle mass in the human body than women. Therefore, for women, getting and preserving muscle is very important to efficient hydration and metabolic function.

Many scientists think the fuzzy, unfocused feeling you experience when you're even mildly parched is your brain's way of saying, "Hey—give me some water!" Put simply, it's an immediate and effective way for your body to tell you your water stores are running low. In fact, research shows that neurons in the brain are able to sense the early warning signs of dehydration—and when they do, they fire off to other neurons and brain regions that regulate mood, putting this internal alarm system in place.

Even more serious, we have seen early studies that link chronic dehydration to the development of Alzheimer's disease. We now know that Alzheimer's and diabetes have a shared pathology, and many doctors are even calling Alzheimer's "type 3 diabetes."[13] Some of the causal links include insulin resistance, inflammation, oxidative stress, obesity, and metabolic syndrome. We believe hydration is the first step in protecting against all these things!

Dr. Simon Thornton, a professor of neuroscience at the University of Lorraine in France, agrees with us. He believes that chronic low-grade dehydration is one of the principal causes behind the development of obesity, diabetes, hypertension, and even Alzheimer's disease.[14] Now, if this were the case, then depleted hydration (hypovolemia) contributes to less brain volume and function.[15] This theory of dehydration is supported further by work showing that total body water decreases with age[16] as well as with increasing body mass index.[17] This suggests that aged and/or obese and/or diabetic patients could be chronically dehydrated. Furthermore, the majority of medications used to treat cardiovascular disease block the very ability of the cells to hydrate. In other words, these drugs are turning off our bodies' ability to activate a system that keeps hydration where we need it most.[18] High blood pressure levels have been associated with brain volume decreases.[19] All of this adds support to the new paradigm of dehydration-induced pathology.

Hydration and Injury Prevention and Concussion

Hydration is mentioned nowhere on the Centers for Disease Control website on its "Brain Injury Safety Tips and Prevention" page. Nor is hydration mentioned on the Mayo Clinic website in the discussion of concussions. We are on a mission to change that, as we believe good and proper hydration is first-line therapy for prevention of many conditions, including concussions (known as mild traumatic brain injury, TBI for short). This is such an important issue, especially as it relates to kids and sports.

Your brain has the consistency of gelatin. It's cushioned from everyday jolts and bumps by cerebrospinal fluid inside your skull. A violent blow to your head and neck or upper body can cause your brain to slam back and forth against the inner walls of your skull. Sudden acceleration or deceleration, caused by a sudden collision or fall, for example, also can cause brain injury. More water means more cushioning and protection.

Mild TBI is a huge burden on our emergency rooms.[20] In the last ten years there has been more than a 100 percent (and in some age groups more than a 200 percent) increase in ER visits related to concussion from sports-related injuries.

MIT researcher Dr. Stephanie Seneff and her colleagues make a very strong case, in an article published in *Surgical Neurology International*,[21] that the rise in sports-related concussions may be related to pre-existing diminished brain resilience due to pervasive environmental toxins and deficient nutrients in athletes. These conditions lead to an "increased susceptibility to what would previously be considered innocuous concussions" and reflect the body's inability to regain equilibrium. Hydration under these new conditions becomes critical for protection and for providing water's number one function: maintaining homeostasis.

CTE and Hydration

Repeated and long-term TBI, when not given enough time to recover, can lead to devastating consequences. You may remember this horrific story from 2011: News of famed hockey player Derek Boogaard's death of apparent overdose at the young age of twenty-eight shocked the sports world. An enforcer on the ice for such teams as the Minnesota Wild and the New York Rangers, he had became a long-time fan favorite for his fighting prowess and intimidation on the ice, which afforded him the nickname "the Boogeyman." But years of knocks to the head and concussions had led him to taking prescription drugs, and while he continued to win on the ice, aggressively playing the game, Boogaard became increasingly moody, erratic, forgetful, and antisocial. When he died, friends and family initially chalked it up to years of drug abuse and wild living catching up to him. But the autopsy report showed a different picture: Boogaard had died of chronic traumatic encephalopathy, also known as CTE, a sister disease to Alzheimer's and known to be caused by repeated blows to the head. It is hard to diagnose and can only be detected posthumously, but what really shocked the coroner was how advanced Boogaard's CTE was. To see that sort of progression of the disease—more advanced than in any other former NHL player who had died from it—at such a young age was stunning. Yet, even though Boogaard's diagnosis made a lot of headlines, the National Hockey League has not acknowledged any link between hockey and the head injuries resulting in CTE that come with playing the game. The good news is that recently the National Football League has donated millions of dollars to University of North Carolina at Chapel Hill to fund research in active rehabilitation strategies in athletes suffering from concussions.[22]

Participants who sustain a concussion can temporarily lose consciousness; feel confused, dizzy, nauseated, and fatigued; and have slurred speech, concentration and sleep problems, irritability and/or depression, and sensitivity to light, to name a few. These symptoms can be seen immediately after injury, or they may come to light hours, days, or even years after the injury. Once you have sustained a mild TBI, you are more at risk for sustaining another.[23] The doctor can diagnose a concussion based on these symptoms with or without the help of imaging such as an MRI or a CT scan. What can confound the diagnosis, though, is dehydration, which can present similarly. Therefore it is important for the athlete to practice excellent hydration skills and for the doctor to make sure the patient is properly hydrated *before evaluating* for a concussion. We draw attention to this important fact for those doctors who are reading this.

In their groundbreaking article mentioned earlier, Dr. Seneff and her colleagues conclude that sports-related concussion is a modern-day problem prompted by diminished brain resilience and relates causality to the following list, all of which the Quench program addresses and why smoothies are such a great pre-sports drink:

- Pesticide and chemical exposure
- Reduced exposure to natural sunlight
- Poor omega 3:6 ratio in diet
- Overconsumption of processed foods[24]

While most major health resources, like the Mayo Clinic website, never mention hydration as a *treatment* for concussion, we believe the Quench program is an excellent adjunct to getting plenty of rest when nursing a brain injury back to health.[25]

Chronic Pain

At least one in five people suffer from chronic pain—and far more experience periodic pain. Dehydration can actually be at the root of some pain—think migraine and muscle cramps—so for these issues, drinking water can be both balm and cure. But even in more complex pain cases, such as acute injury, joint aches, and menstrual cramps, hydration can help. Research shows that dehydration makes the pain you're experiencing feel worse.[26] It makes sense. When you're dehydrated, water is rerouted: Instead of heading to your tissues and joints, it heads straight to your brain, heart, and other vital organs that need water in order to keep you alive. That can make tissues and joints stiffer, cause waste by-products such as lactic acid to build up, and contribute to pain-causing inflammation, too.

What's more, dehydration increases brain activity linked to pain—whereas adequate hydration calms that activity, leading to lower pain levels.[27] That may be why many functional medicine doctors recommend *extra* hydration, sometimes in the form of intravenous fluids, to patients with fibromyalgia. Simply getting hydration levels up to an optimal level helps ease the all-over agony and fatigue of this chronic condition.

DR. DANA'S CASE STUDY

Betty

When Betty first arrived in my office, her fibromyalgia was so severe that she couldn't work. A fifty-four-year-old woman living in Nantucket, she explained that "everything hurt," so much so that she had two to four glasses of wine at night to cope with the pain and her inability to fall asleep. The wine helped her pass out—but she couldn't sleep through the night.

Not surprisingly, Betty was depressed and overweight. She had come to see me about bio-identical hormone replacement for her menopausal symptoms. By the end of our appointment, it was clear to me that we needed to address far more than hot flashes. I suggested she try the Quench program and drastically cut her alcohol intake. Eager to make a change in her life, she agreed.

Three weeks later, Betty practically bounced into my office. "Dr. Cohen, I feel *so much better*!" she told me. Today (one year later), she describes herself as a new person: Instead of alcohol, she sips water and smoothies. She's changed her diet, and she has started exercising after thinking that her fibromyalgia made it impossible for her to do so. She experienced a drastic reduction in pain and an increase in energy for the first time in decades. The Quench program with its small shifts was the impetus she needed to get to those larger changes. She was able to give up alcohol altogether, which she no longer needed to mask the pain, and in turn her sleeping improved.

Sleep

Not sleeping as deeply or as long as you'd like? Join the club. Nearly half of all Americans don't get enough shut-eye in any given week.[28] But popping a pill isn't a long-term solution, and sleep aids come with all sorts of risks. Skip the meds, and choose water instead. Hydration offers several basic sleep benefits. For starters, it keeps your mouth and nasal passages moist, which reduces sleep-disrupting snoring. Adequate hydration can also prevent leg cramps, which can wake you, even if you don't remember it the next day. Even if you're not prone to sawing logs or waking up with a charley horse, drinking water during the day is important for sleeping better at night.

Why might this be? There's a big—and largely under-explored—answer at play. Most of our body's detoxification takes place while you're unconscious. And water is at the heart of that detoxification process. That's why sleep is so restorative: You literally wake up with a cleaner, more effective operating system. New research shows that when you're asleep, your body increases movement of several key fluids, including cerebrospinal and interstitial fluid, in your brain, spine, lymph system, and other key areas. This increase in fluid movement helps your body and brain clear certain metabolites and toxins, such as beta amyloid protein, which contributes to Alzheimer's disease. The better hydrated you are, the better the process works.[29, 30, 31]

Fortunately, sleeping better doesn't require drinking two liters of water before you hit the hay. (See the sidebar on urination for more on why daytime hydration doesn't have to sabotage your night.) If you're drinking water and choosing hydrating foods throughout the day, you're doing enough to help your system detoxify and get deep, restorative sleep. Still worried about 1 a.m. bathroom runs? Refrain from drinking more than a half cup of liquid for about an hour before bed—and skip the nightcap, too. In addition to being dehydrating, alcohol is a sleep disruptor and bladder irritant.

What about bathroom breaks?

Yes, drinking enough water is going to send you to the bathroom more often—and that's a good thing. You should be going at least every three hours, and some doctors (like holistic doctor Gabriel Cousens, MD, author of *Spiritual Nutrition*) even say every two hours. Chances are, you along with the rest of modern society spend far too much time seated. Getting up to walk to the bathroom is an easy way to get your blood and oxygen pumping and enable you to fight back against the many ill effects of a sedentary lifestyle.

Urination itself gets a bad rap, but it's actually one of the best things you can do for your bladder and kidneys: Every time you urinate, you clear out lingering bacteria, waste by-products, and other compounds that go through your body's "filtering" system.

You may be wondering how you can pee eight times or more a day—yet go seven to nine hours without doing so at night. You have your brain to thank for that. As you slumber, it releases an antidiuretic hormone (ADH) that helps your kidneys concentrate urine instead of overfilling your bladder and rousing you with that tingling, I've-got-to-go-now feeling. That's also why your urine can look so dark in the morning; it's ultraconcentrated.

As you age, your body makes less ADH, which is why so many older people wake to urinate throughout the night when they didn't do so earlier in their life. It's also why it's key to use the bathroom right before you turn in for the night, at any age. You'll want to make sure you're not saving most of your water intake for right before bed—and if you're hydrating throughout the day, you won't feel like you need to. If you're practicing good sleep hygiene and front-loading your water intake, yet still find you have to wake throughout the night to use the bathroom, try avoiding alcohol and too much caffeine, and seek out your doctor's help. You could also try a teaspoon of ground chia seeds in a half cup of tea about an hour before bed. For some, that recipe acts like a sponge to hold urine in longer during sleep.

Cancer

No, water alone can't cure cancer. But emerging research shows that hydration can play a key role in reducing the risk of several common forms of the disease. Italian researchers found that adults who drank less water were more likely to get bladder and lower urinary tract cancer. They speculate that increasing water helps push carcinogens through your urinary tract. The less contact these harmful substances have with your tissues, the less likely they are to cause cancer.[32]

The same team of Italian researchers found that increased water intake may reduce the risk of colorectal cancer. While the regions may be different, the mechanism is the same: Water helps stool pass more quickly through the colon and rectum, the last six inches of your large intestine, thereby limiting these areas' contact with carcinogens that you get from your diet or the environment.

Weight Loss

Hydration is essential to weight loss. We mentioned earlier that a 2010 study showed that drinking water before every meal can help you lose five pounds in just three months. Other studies have shown similar results. While researchers often thank a reduction in calorie intake for this phenomenon—water fills up your stomach, which makes it harder to overeat—it may turn off hunger pangs, too. And water has no caloric value. When you substitute water for other drinks that have few nutrients and, even worse, are usually sweetened with offenders like high-fructose corn syrup or sucrose, you naturally reduce the added calories.

But there are other mechanisms at play. A 2010 study from Vanderbilt University found that water increases activity in the sympathetic nervous system, which actually causes your body to burn more calories. In fact, researchers say drinking even three sixteen-ounce glasses of water a day increases calorie burning enough to help you drop five pounds in a year without making any other changes to your lifestyle.[33] A similar study from German researchers found that drinking a sixteen-ounce glass of water boosted metabolic rate 30 percent—that's an average of two hundred extra calories a day.[34]

All this aside, when you choose water, you're *not* choosing other beverages that can contribute to weight gain, like sugary sodas, calorie-laden coffee drinks, alcoholic beverages, and even artificially sweetened drinks—especially diet soda, which research has repeatedly linked to weight gain as well as a host of health problems[35] like osteoporosis, stroke, and dementia.[36]

EMERGING SCIENCE IN WATER RESEARCH

Water is a slippery subject. Though we know a lot about the properties of water, there is also so much we don't know. As scientists continue to try to understand the elusive molecule, research about water and cell efficiency is emerging from laboratories around the world. Water science at the molecular level has the scientific community abuzz, and it's shaping our understanding of how water functions, and more relevant for you, it is the basis of *Quench*.

This new science reveals that the water in our cells is a *different type* of water: the same kind of water we can find in plants. We already know that water exists as a liquid, a gas, or a solid, but new findings are uncovering a fourth, gel-like state of water, just 10 percent more viscous than the liquid state. This change in water phases takes place at the molecular level. We can't see the molecular change with our naked eye, but in this state, water hydrates more efficiently. For you, it means you can *drink less liquid, yet be more hydrated.* While we cannot yet exactly measure how much more efficient this gel-like water is, we can surmise it to be substantial, extrapolating from desert and in extremis environments, where this form of hydration has been in use since ancient times.

Global Ancient Strategies

Some of our best clues about what foods hydrate effectively come from extreme environments where access to abundant water is limited. Here is where we most see humans turning to foods to supplement their water sources and hydration needs. Besides our stories from actual deserts, other in extremis environments that demand human adaptation are high-altitude regions such as those in the Himalayas and the Peruvian highlands.

Archeological and forensic analysis of ancient pottery from Hualcayan in the High Andes show surprising evidence that stews were the staple form of hydration. They included gelatins released by grains. Anthropologist Dr. Rebecca Bria states, "By interpreting my microbotanical information with botanical analysis we actually found 'gelatinized' starches embedded in the pottery."[37]

Food scientist Harold McGee, writing on the science and molecular characteristics of food in his 1984 book *On Food and Cooking*, notes that heating starch grains in the presence of water breaks down the crystalline layers and causes the starches to gelatinize, or form a viscous complex with water. These grain-released gelatins further enhanced the absorptive and therefore hydrating power of the cooking water found in stews.

Indeed, these ancient strategies of changing the hydrating power of water by adding plants such as grains, herbs, seeds, or roots were deployed throughout the ages, on all continents. Overwhelming evidence resides in ethnographic and medieval records showing plants were used for hydration and the purification of water. Slow-cooked stews and pottages released more gelatin, changing the molecular structure of the cooking liquid. Beers and meads accomplished the same change through fermentation and were globally used strategies to further purify, or replace entirely, contaminated or tainted waters.

NEW STATES OF WATER

These new states or phases of water are being discussed at some of the world's most prestigious institutions. Studies that support this are hot off the press, confirming previously unrecognized states of water.

In the summer of 2017, Katrin Amann-Winkel, working in her laboratory at the University of Stockholm, identified a different and new phase of water. She saw that it "transforms into a viscous liquid which almost immediately transforms to a different, even more viscous, liquid of much lower density than ice."[38] Laura Maestro and her fellow scientists at Oxford University also confirm that water switches between states.[39] Maestro has said, "The existence of these two states in liquid water plays an important role in biological systems."

The important takeaway here is that a new state of water is critical to molecular function—with newfound consequences for how our body runs. This different state of water is more organized, and the organized molecules become more effective at their work, like an orchestra with a conductor. Far more efficient than musicians playing without coherence. This emerging science is so new that the scientific community hasn't yet settled on what to call this new phase of water. It has been called **structured water**, **gel** or **EZ water**, **liquid crystalline**, or **ordered** or **coherent water**. Throughout the book we mostly call it gel or structured water.

The Saykally Group at the University of California, Berkeley is using ultrafast laser spectroscopy to investigate one single water molecule, and their findings also show that water exists in other states besides liquid, gas, and solid. As an important aside, R. J. Saykally, lead author of the study, notes, "Water is the most important substance on the planet. Its unique and versatile hydrogen bond network underlies many of the processes responsible for life as we know it. Yet, and despite centuries of study, vital questions regarding the intrinsic nature of water remain unanswered."[40]

A research group from Cornell University has found that water forms a "spine of hydration" around DNA. Lars Petersen, lead author of the study, states, "New results give very strong support to a picture where water at room temperature can't decide in which of the two forms it should be, high or low density, which results in local fluctuations between the two. Water is not a complicated liquid, but two simple liquids with a complicated relationship." Petersen concludes that "a change in the hydration state can lead to dramatic changes to the DNA structure." As you can see, scientists are agreeing that something unusual and not discussed before is going on with the water molecule, and it is not so simple as simple H_2O.

STRUCTURED WATER

The most exciting emerging science in recent years is the work coming out of the laboratory of Dr. Gerald Pollack, who first indisputably identified, with documented experiments, this new gel state of water. Dr. Pollack, from the University of Washington Seattle, holds a PhD in bioengineering. With thirty years of experiments behind him, he is revered by a global following.

Pollack's laboratory experiments identified what he calls EZ water, which stands for "exclusionary zone" water, alluding to its ability to eliminate all particles within this zone.

In gel water's "exclusionary zone," Dr. Pollack saw that water molecules can begin to stick or cohere and squeeze out any molecules larger than their own. Remember that water molecules are among the tiniest in the world, and they filter out other, larger, but still minuscule particles, including those of toxins and other unwanted substances. No one had actually seen this occur until Dr. Pollack found a way to show it in his lab. In the denser gel form, or EZ phase, molecules coalesce to squeeze out or exclude any larger particles. EZ water is, simply put, water filtering itself.

Exclusion zone water, according to Dr. Pollack, has *vitally important differences* from plain liquid water, H_2O. It is denser and has more oxygen. But here is the most surprising difference: While liquid water has a charge that is neutral, EZ water has a negative charge. Though a negative charge may sound negative, it is actually how water forms a battery and begins producing and storing energy inside us—the very energy we need to move, think, heal, and repair. This water is not only denser but also better able to conduct all our electrical functions. These experiments measured the amount of electromagnetic force, or the increased energy, in the water.

WHY GEL WATER ACTS AS IT DOES

Our favorite story about how all this got started comes from Dr. Pollack himself. While examining a heart muscle cell, he pierced the cellular wall and noticed that the water inside the cell didn't leak out. It didn't even drip out. He wondered: Why, when you break open the cell membrane, does the water stay inside? "That water must be different, funny," he realized.

He started asking around, and he learned that no one else really knew why either. Pursuing this question eventually led to Pollack convening the international Conference on the Physics, Biology and Chemistry of Water, now in its twelfth year, where scientists and thinkers go to explore current theories of the behavior of water and search for new answers. Although water is generally thought of as having a diluting effect, this new research shows that it can be cohesive as well. Dr. Pollack's breakthrough work came when he noticed how different water was when its molecules linked up over time and across space. Together they became more and more tightly knit—they were not yet stationary ice crystals, like snowflakes, but rather overlapping or interlinked crystals, much like lace or crocheted netting but still in a fluid state. This is also known as a liquid crystalline state. They form not a solitary H_2O connection but a more complex one, H_3O_2. These findings are still embroiled in controversy; after all, water has been thought of as simply H_2O for a very long time, but it is promising, and many scientists agree it can now explain how water functions in nature.

Also, as we said earlier, there is an increasing consensus that water exists in phases other than liquid, vapor, and ice. A Harvard University research group concluded in 2008 that water inside cellular proteins is different from liquid water and forms an ordered hexagonal shape that comes in many sheets or layers. This is a description strikingly similar to EZ water structure.[41]

What we can glean from Pollack and the other studies is that water is sophisticated, more sophisticated than we thought. Water was never just a background material, not just a universal solvent, but *the* major activator of chemical and electrical ignition. In this molecular world, water is a *vibrating continuum*, sliding in and out of phases and forms, while appearing to our naked eye to be . . . just water. When liquid slips into the gel state, and we will show you how it does this, it amplifies water's life-giving properties. The most important things you need to know about this amazing new science of water is that there exists a water that is denser, activated by light waves, and has more measurable energy. We are still figuring out how this works, but it could hint at accelerating our cells' ability to repair, regenerate, and, ultimately, provide more vitality.

WHERE STRUCTURED WATER IS FOUND

Gel water exists in all living cells, even plants. We can *taste* and *feel* the difference. Gel water can seem as thin as liquid but slightly silkier, and it can expand to become as thick as gelatin. It is in all sorts of foods. For example, that much maligned iceberg lettuce is really a superhydrating food. The water inside the lettuce is structured. And it is gel water in bone broth that everyone finds so healing. When you soak chia seeds, you actually see the gel forming.

This answers the question: How exactly does gel water hydrate differently from regular water? As far as we know now, and there is yet so much to discover, gel water hydrates differently because it is a different stage of water, one that not only moistens longer but conducts electrical function in the body far more efficiently. A great example is when doctors apply a gel to the skin to get a better reading from ultrasound and electrocardiogram tests. This is because denser gel is a great conductor. Electrical conduction has to do with all those electrolytes you hear about, which are minerals, abundantly found in plants. When dissolved in water, they release their electrical charge. Because density and charge matter a great deal to efficient conduction, gel water conducts electricity very efficiently. A lot. More energy, less fatigue, more healing power. This is to say that if we faithfully eat fresh fruits and veggies, we are getting a power-packed food that has more measureable energy and more hydrating capacity than a bottle of water.

Desert Cowboys Pack Herbs

To hydrate well on a diet mostly of beef, the famed nomadic cowboys—gauchos—of the Uruguayan pampa plains used yerba maté, an intense herbal infusion made from a type of holly tree. These infusions were rich in plant nutrients and minerals, and, as evidenced by the gauchos' robust health in such arid conditions, delivered optimal hydration. Yerba maté has been extensively studied in the 1960s by the Pasteur Institute in Paris, which concluded, "It is difficult to find a plant in any area of the world equal to this herb in nutritional value, containing practically all the vitamins necessary to sustain life." Another study revealed that yerba maté contains a very high content of mineral elements and the right balance of electrolytes. We now have some evidence that yerba maté contributes to weight balance and even weight loss.[42]

One thing is certainly clear: Plants are packed with nutrients, many of which can only be released in the solvent action of water molecules. So by the solvency of water, plants deliver nutrients to our bodies *in addition* to the hydrating water they hold.

WE ARE TRULY SOLAR POWERED

Hydration, ironically, starts with the sun. The relationship between sun and water is original and originating. Hydration happens when sunlight hits the water molecules, even through our skin. Dr. Pollack proposes that when the light waves reach water, even inside us at the cellular level, the water molecule splits, resulting in a more negative charge, turning water into an energizing battery. Batteries hold and store electrical charge to be used for energy, and cells do this as well. *Sun and water together turn us into batteries.* Sunlight and infrared light and all the spectrums in between determine our energy and the quality of our hydration. In addition to food, sunlight is the most natural, most accessible way to help our cells function. Exposure to light, whether in the form of visible light or infrared (the light you can't see) helps build, or literally grow, gel water inside the body. According to Pollack, "The energy for building water structure comes from the sun. Radiant energy from wavelengths, ranging from ultraviolet through visible to infrared, converts ordinary bulk or liquid water into ordered water." Through his experiments, he shows that water absorbs light energy freely from the environment and uses that energy to build EZ water. Additional energy input, whether from the sun or food from plants, creates additional EZ buildup.

This is why Pollack describes this fourth phase of water with a different chemical equation. In EZ water, electrons share a negative and a positive charge to make this new H_3O_2. "Absorbed radiant energy splits water molecules; the negative moiety constitutes the building block of the EZ, while the positive moiety binds with water molecules to form free hydronium ions (H_3O^+), which diffuse throughout the water. Adding additional light (radiant energy) stimulates more charge separation," thus building more structured water.[43]

Dr. Pollack isn't the only person looking at how light is used for energy in the body. In fact, a new study has recently come out in 2014 integrating the role of light water and plants inside mammals. This recent study, published in the *Journal of Cell Science*, documents how the chlorophyll molecule inside the body works with light to produce ATP, which is a molecule that stores our cells' energy.[44] For the first time the authors show that ingested plant molecules, inside a mammal's body, take light and produce energy in the form of ATP. Sound familiar? Like photosynthesis in plants, they propose that through eating green plants (chlorophyll), mammals are able to derive energy from sunlight.

When light passes through skin, it starts a chain reaction in all cells, and that chain reaction passes along the charge and gives us energy. Think of the phrase "I need to recharge my batteries"—it's like plugging in our phone or computer—we are recharging with our light source, and that charge is conducted by a well-hydrated body.

Besides exposure to light to continue to build this gel water inside the body, you also want to *eat foods* that contain this structured water. This also helps build electrical charge. One kind of food is water squeezed from plants. When you juice or blend, you squeeze structured water from plants. As Pollack notes, "You're putting into your body what your body really needs. From my point of view, this is the biggest revolution in medicine. Just by drinking the right kind of water, you can really improve your health and even reverse pathology."

CONNECTING THE DOTS

This new science can mean accumulating gains for our hydration, enhancing our health and vibrancy in challenging times. Better hydration will create better function, protecting all our systems and tissues. Dehydration is harming us. Now more than ever we are all suffering from our artificial environments. But just in time, new science has identified a different phase of water, found both inside our cells and inside plant cells as well. We can easily improve our cell function by maintaining and improving gel volume from all-natural sources. We can incorporate hydrating foods into our diet to create more energy. Our Quench plan delivers this new science to you through our simple smoothie recipes to hydrate all the way to the cellular level, just as we live in ever more dehydrating conditions.

CHAPTER 2

Eat Your Water

Food for Optimal Hydration

No water. no life. No blue, no green.

—*Sylvia Earle*

Did you know that your food can suck hydration out of you? Or, conversely, rehydrate you? Rehydrate you even more profoundly than water alone? For example, an apple with a bottle of water hydrates more than two bottles of water. Here's how that works: The fibrous materials in that apple serve as a sponge to help hold the moisture inside itself longer, and longer inside you.

But before we even start discussing food, we want to talk about change. Change is what we are made for, growth and adaptability; it's the most common human quality, it's in your ancestry, and yours to claim. Your food choices can put an end to some of our modern fatigue—a lot of it, actually. But we have to leave behind our old way of eating. If you haven't changed your food habits in a while, it's time to. It's time to eat your water.

Why? We truly are in a new environment. Our current living patterns, including our grab-and-go foods, wipe us out. They create excessive weariness and, most important, squelch our joy. The reason to get hydrated, and use food to do it, is ultimately a joyful one: It's to receive more life. More liveliness. Higher cognitive function and appreciation. And coupling water with food turns out to be the absolute smartest strategy on the planet, one designed by nature. Where did separating hydration and food into two categories even happen? Nature packaged them together into one superefficient delivery system.

Tricks for Avoiding Environmental Dehydration

Problem: Heat dehydrates. Think of all those lights and electronic devices that warm up by just being on. Have you ever noticed how hot your computer can get, or even your phone?

Quench Trick: Keep your phones and computers in low blue-light mode—it's cooler. Better yet, walk away from your electronics for five minutes every hour. Work in natural daylight as much as you can. Consider bringing a nice desk lamp to your office and turning off overhead lights. Take your meetings outside for a walk. A safe perimeter for cell phone use is two feet. Keep your cell phone two feet away from your body and use an earpiece—or better yet, use the speakerphone when you can.

Problem: All that sitting and slumping over keyboards and phones suppresses and restricts the vital flow of fluid throughout our whole system.

Quench Trick: Get in a little movement and check in with your posture in each hour. Slouching? Shoulders down, chest up. Doesn't that feel better?

Problem: Air-conditioning may seem like it helps with heat, and it does—but it still dehydrates by pulling humidity out of the room. Building materials like carpets, synthetic curtains, furniture, and sealed environments all conspire to suck up vapor in the air. Take a good look around your room or office and notice all the things there that compete with you to absorb the little humidity available indoors.

Quench Trick: We can compensate for these environments by rehumidifying. But humidifying a whole room can require expensive equipment. An easy fix is to have a small diffuser near you, so you are humidifying your body and not the whole room. Even simple things like putting an open jar of water on our desk or adding plants where we work or in our homes make a difference we can feel.

Adding essential oils to a diffuser brings in aromatic plant molecules, an ingenious but often unrecognized way to receive hydration. And the vapor goes to your nasal passages and lungs, and, yes, that is a form of soothing hydration right there. A simple trick, when at the office or in meetings, is to keep a nice cup of tea near you and inhale the vapors a little here and there, even if you don't drink that cup.

Problem: Cars, planes, trains, and even subways are dehydrating capsules. They are some of the most dehumidified environments around, with airplanes winning hands down. A healthy indoor humidity is between 50 and 60 percent, but airplanes can have less than 20 percent humidity, sometimes dropping down to as low as 1 percent. Cars are tough, too: For every hour you spend in a car, you reduce your hydration by exchanging moist air for dry, deoxygenated air. Dehydration from travel can accelerate stiffness and deflate skin, the result of all that sitting with very little motion while in a dehumidified environment.

Quench Trick: Never travel without something to drink in your car, open the windows intermittently to bring fresh air inside the car, and practice micromovements at stoplights.

Problem: A lack of sunlight indoors, in our homes and offices, is costing us our hydration in ways we never suspected. Not only are we living high-stress lives in intentionally dehumidified rooms, we are out of natural sunlight, which has so much to do with our hydration as well as warming us and calming our whole nervous system.

Quench Trick: Become alert to your need for sunlight, and take ten-to-fifteen-minute breaks outdoors and bask in the open air on your lunch hour. We can't yet say how much sunlight everybody should get, because every body probably needs different exposure, but those few lunch-hour minutes should treat you well (subject of course to your doctor's clearance, if you have issues). You can benefit from light waves even on cloudy days. Finally, new evidence is coming in fast that we need information from sunlight to set our inner clocks appropriately each day. That first hour of daylight may turn out to be far more crucial than we knew.

Problem: Stress and pressure created by our busy modern lives drive neurochemicals into our systems that require our bodies to do way more work, again drawing on our water reserves to process.

Quench Trick: Smoothies and hydrating foods send protective nutrients in to help buffer us. A regular habit of deep breaths resets our system and draws hydrating air further in.

In our Quench program, we have put what nature intended back together again. It will just take a little adapting on your part—but isn't that what we do? And we give easy shifts to accomplish that. After all, we are just asking you to add in some smart smoothies, get drinks at key points of the day, and add hydrating food to compensate when you do eat something dehydrating. Can it be any simpler than that?

For example, if you reach for two apples instead of two slices of pizza...okay, unlikely, but how about one slice of pizza and one apple? You've just rebalanced your body's inner calculations about how to spend energy digesting. Your body knows it's going to get hydrating help from that apple. And you've just recharged your battery on the spot by taking in the electrical charge that comes with gel water from that apple.

In this chapter we give you the information to change yourself. Quench enables you to change your food choices with understanding, results, and pleasure. We give you energizing, can-do tips and techniques in our plan.

WATER IS NOT JUST BLUE; IT'S GREEN

Maybe this is the first time you have heard of using food as water. We haven't generally thought of water as nutritious; rather, we think of it as functional, as moistening, as wet. And you've had it drummed into you that hydration requires eight glasses a day, or half your body weight in ounces. Indeed, the widely known eight-glasses-a-day recommendation has been traced to original government recommendations, which gave hydration guidelines based on total ounces.[1] The surprise is that in those original guidelines, 45 percent of those ounces came from *food*. Over the years urban legend has morphed it into ounces from *liquids* only, and finally *water* only. But getting our hydration from water *and* food turns out to be the absolute smartest strategy on the planet, one designed by nature. Nature packaged them together into one superefficient delivery system.

> **I heard that drinking half my body weight in water (in ounces) is what I am supposed to be doing—is this true?**
>
> Drinking half your body weight in water in ounces is a general guideline that is widely used, because it is an easy one. For example, under these guidelines a 120-pound woman would drink sixty

ounces of water per day. It's not a bad guideline, but it's far from gospel. In reality, hydration is sensitive to many conditions, not just your body weight. You may be in dry conditions, you may be young, in shape, or have medications you are taking, each requiring different hydration calibrations. Or you may be older and have less muscle (your body's biggest holder of hydration); you may be sweating a lot; but above all, what you eat makes a big difference in adequate hydration.

In *Quench*, we ask that you pay attention to your own signals for drinking, not some set amount. Our top two signals are fatigue, especially the afternoon crash, and brain fog. Right behind those are headaches, stiffness and joint pain, irritability, and low mood. Dry tongue or throat and dry nasal passages are early signals, too. We recommend you hydrate more efficiently by loading hydration early in your day, and include many juicy fruits and veggies that provide fiber to help keep you hydrated longer.

Ranging between 80 to 98 percent water by volume, plants are the perfect biological packaging. The next time you bite into an apple or a pear, think about how that fruit is giving you water that is not only pure, or purer, but deeply hydrating, and full of nutrition and minerals to boot. Its genius is in its design-by-nature package of nutrients and hydration in perfect functional balance. Not too much, not too little, nutrient rich, fiber rich, and full of water. Anytime you eat a plant—whether it's a leafy green, a pear, or even chia seeds—it is a form of water.

Top 12 Hydrating Veggies (percent water)	Top 12 Hydrating Fruits (percent water)
1. Cucumbers 96.7%	1. Starfruit 91.4%
2. Romaine lettuce 95.6%	2. Watermelon 91.4%
3. Celery 95.4%	3. Strawberries 91%
4. Radishes 95.3%	4. Grapefruit 90.5%
5. Zucchini 95%	5. Cantaloupe 90.2%
6. Tomatoes 94.5%	6. Pineapple 87%
7. Peppers 93.9%	7. Raspberries 87%
8. Cauliflower 92.1%	8. Blueberries 85%
9. Spinach 91.4%	9. Kiwi 84.2%
10. Broccoli 90.7%	10. Apples 84%
11. Carrots 90%	11. Pears 84%
12. Sprouts 86.5%	12. Grapes 81.5%

There is no denying it—water-rich foods are also nutrient rich, packed with antioxidants, proteins and their amino acids, minerals, and vitamins. They also carry nutrients like calcium, magnesium, potassium, and sodium, which, activated by the electrical charge in water, are then known as electrolytes. But what our new science has alerted us to is that water, full of those electrolytes, is also *full of electrons* that run our electrical function. Water conducts electricity, not only for fuel but for cognition, judgment, and mood. Remember that the quality of our hydration has everything to do with the quality of electrical conduction. We can't say it enough: Water conducts electricity, and hydration runs our electrical function.

This shifts water from being simply wet, simply moistening, or even just cleansing, to being fuel. And get this: Because of the fiber in plants, the water stays in our system longer because we absorb it more slowly. It's a triple play of health: pure water, absorbent fiber, and not only needed nutrients but electrolytes. *Because of these multiple effects, we believe plants hydrate more efficiently than a glass of plain water alone.*

How Cows Hydrate

Cows are out there grazing on that 97 percent water-laden grass all day, staying moist. Granted, they still need to drink, but that fab combo of water-rich, lush grass plus the digested fibers that retain moisture goes a long way to cover their hydration. Contrast that with grain-fed cows that we know need to drink more water and are nutritionally inferior.

Grazing cows drink less water. Measurements made in the summer of 2009 at the Save Your Dairy Farm in Arizona noted that their herd of 130 grass-fed cows drank on average around 1,800 gallons of water per day. But a similarly sized herd of grain-fed cows would consume about 3,000 to 4,000 gallons per day.[2]

At the time of publication of this book, as yet unpublished studies are hinting that plants may be twice as hydrating as a glass of water; imagine that!

FOLLOW THE PIZZA

Remember earlier we talked about pizza and an apple? Why did we replace one slice of pizza with an apple? Because pizza is dehydrating. How does that exactly work?

The easy answer is that pizza is laden with the wrong kind of salt, which makes you lose more fluid than you take in, and your body doesn't have enough water and other fluids to carry out its normal functions. If you don't replace lost fluids, of course you'll get dehydrated.

The long answer is that our cells use and store water in two compartments: the intracellular fluid (ICF) and the extracellular fluid (ECF). The ICF holds about 60 to 65 percent of the body water inside the cell, and the ECF holds about 35 to 40 percent water surrounding the cell. The nutrients, such as chloride, potassium, magnesium, and sodium, help keep the ICF and ECF levels balanced. If any molecule becomes too concentrated in one compartment, it will pull water from the other to dilute itself.

Back to the pizza: The sodium from the tomato sauce and cheese—and the pepperoni or other salty toppings—accumulates in the ECF, which pulls water from the ICF. This sends signals to the brain that the cell is dehydrating. The brain signals you to drink more water. In fact, bloating results from just this imbalance.

SALT: A HYDRATING SOLUTION

Wait—salt can *help* you stay hydrated?

We just explained how sodium (aka salt) is dehydrating. It's true that an excessive amount of common *processed* table salt isn't good for you. Your kidneys use water to filter salt and flush it from your system in the form of urine. It's a normal, everyday process. But if you're already running low on water—and your diet is chock-full of added processed sodium—this combination can lead to dehydration and eventually kidney problems.

Skimping on salt isn't the solution, though. In fact, it may be harmful to your health. Sodium is a key electrolyte. With the help of potassium, sodium is required to balance your body's internal electrical charge. Sodium and potassium dissolving in water drive an essential cellular function actually called the sodium-potassium cellular pump. In our bodies, sodium provides positively charged ions, while potassium provides negatively charged ions, and this combination generates electrical charges in your cell membranes. It's a constant back-and-forth process that keeps cells—including your nerves and neurotransmitters—functioning. If you don't have enough salt in your system, your body's internal charge isn't balanced, and your cells can't receive and transmit impulses the way they should. A small amount of natural salt is absolutely essential for hydration.

That's why you often see everyday exercisers as well as professional athletes chugging on sports drinks during and after competition. They're not just replenishing the water they've lost; they're also restocking their body's sodium and potassium stores. If you do exercise, skip sports drinks loaded with artificial sweeteners, synthetic chemicals, food coloring, and other unnecessary additives.

Why are sports drinks becoming less popular as a way to hydrate?

Sports drinks and other "hydrating" solutions get a bad rap, and for good reason. Sports drinks are loaded with sugar you never asked for in your "healthy" drinks. After spending the day outside, you just want to sip on something satisfying without the blood sugar spike. Sports drinks are made not only with unwanted sugars or sugar substitutes, they also use synthetic electrolytes—that is, manufactured minerals, not natural ones. And with synthetic minerals, sports drinks lose the broad spectrum of trace minerals, whose work on behalf of hydration is only starting to be understood as important regulators of metabolic function. The same is true for drinks with added vitamins. Those vitamins are synthetic, not natural, and are often full of sugar to enhance taste. Try our natural sports drink recipe in chapter 5

One recent Cochrane review (that's an extensive review of scientific literature, which is considered by many to be the gold standard of scientific evidence in health) actually found that a low-sodium diet increased the production of kidney hormones that can actually *raise* blood pressure. Low-sodium diets have also been shown to raise your levels of catecholamines—those are fight-or-flight neurotransmitters that can speed your heart rate and cause your blood vessels to constrict. Which is to say a low-sodium diet may not be the high blood pressure (hypertension) cure it's been touted as—and may even contribute to hypertension.

THE SODIUM-HYDRATION LINK

When it comes to salt, think quality, not quantity, for optimum hydration and health. Table salt doesn't have the right properties to help hydrate you and keep you healthy. But other healthy salts—that is, natural, minimally processed salt—play a crucial role in hydration. That's because these salts contain more than sodium. They also carry trace minerals like iodine, iron, potassium, magnesium, and calcium. Some of them, including potassium and calcium, are electrolytes that keep your electrical balance in check and your cells functioning healthfully as you add water to your system.

Choose:

- Sea salt
- Celtic salt
- Rock salt
- Himalayan salt

These salts can provide a burst of flavor to your food. But even better, start salting your water instead of your food. Adding a pinch of healthy salt to your glass of water or smoothie is a simple way to make sure you have the ideal electrolyte exchange to keep water balanced inside you.

While we recommend swapping your saltshaker for a healthier form of natural salt, it's worth noting that even regular table salt may not be the health foe experts have spent decades claiming it is. For example, a recent study of more than 2,600 adults at Emory University found that not only was a sodium intake of 1,500 to 2,000 mg per day not associated with a higher risk of heart disease, but those people who were slightly more likely to outlive those who consumed an average of less than 1,500 a day. That's right—sodium was actually tied to a *longer* life. Another French study of more than eight thousand adults found that sodium intake wasn't linked to systolic blood pressure, leading researchers to claim that the link between salt and blood pressure was "overstated." Of course, the French are famed for their use of sea salts.

Hyponatremia

You *can* drink too much water. Water intoxication is dangerous, because it can dilute the sodium in our blood. Compounding that, sodium is also being lost in our sweat. Meanwhile, sodium levels within other cells—in the skin, muscles, and internal organs—remain constant. To correct the imbalance, osmosis draws water out of the extracellular fluid, causing the cells to become engorged. Hands and feet balloon. It doesn't happen often, because our kidneys can produce a large quantity of urine in a brief time period to correct this imbalance of sodium levels. However with athletes, hyponatremia can occur in prolonged endurance events such as a marathon. Symptoms include vomiting, headache, bloating, swollen feet and hands, disorientation, undue fatigue, and wheezy breathing. While the edema from hyponatremia is rare, we believe that excessive water drinking still depletes you of important minerals and electrolytes. It isn't only athletes who need to be cautious; this can happen to Bikram yoga devotees and even kids in after-school sports. That's why we protect you with plant-based drinks.

Most people in fair to good health can handle more than the 1,500 mg of salt daily that many health organizations recommend. But perhaps more important, salt itself may not be the reason some studies link high blood pressure and heart problems to sodium. Instead, it may be that processed food, abundant in processed salt—think fast food and other fried fare, microwave meals, and junk food like chips—is the real culprit.

Dana has suggested to many of her patients over the years to add a pinch of sea salt to a glass of water, especially in the morning. It's tasty, helps keep you hydrated, and it's particularly good for people who have abnormally low blood pressure and those who dehydrate quickly. Make it a routine in your day.

Dehydrating Foods

Foods to limit, avoid, or compensate for:

Alcohol: Alcohol takes a lot of your inner hydration to process. Your strategy here is always to drink a glass of water for every alcoholic beverage you down. It also makes your bar tab cheaper!

Sugar: You need a lot of hydration to process and filter sugar, and that isn't even accounting for the cascading effects of sugar that draw even more on your hydration banks, such as sugar's impact on insulin. If you go for the donut, the ice cream, or the cake (occasionally), then compensate by drinking some extra water. (Also see our "Sweeten the Deal" sidebar in chapter 8.)

Grains, starches, meats, cheeses: Have you ever been knocked comatose after Thanksgiving dinner or a business lunch at a pasta joint that led to an unexpected afternoon nap? An easy fix is to eat a larger portion of salad or soup and a smaller portion of grains, starches, or meats. Remember, we are not asking you to avoid these delicious foods but instead to reduce their portions and compensate with added hydration.

Coffee and teas: If you drink excessive amounts of these beverages, in the four-to-six-cup (eight-ounce) range per day, you will definitely feel the diuretic effects that lead to dehydration. Simply add hot water after cup number two and start diluting as you go. Often it is simply the feel of a comforting warm cup that we are after. You could also whip in a teaspoon of grass-fed butter or ghee—an ancient Himalayan strategy that slows down the impact of caffeine.

MICROBIOMES

Benjamin Franklin is said to have quipped, "In wine there is wisdom, in beer there is freedom, in water there is bacteria."

Ben was right, but he forgot that bacteria can be GOOD for you. If you haven't been following the remarkable new understanding of the need for good bacteria inside of us, just know that microbes, when in balance—*and hydrated*—are literally our closest allies in life. When we drink more water in the form of plants, we are helping our microbiome to do its job by feeding those microbes the nutrients, fiber, and *water* they need. They too need more and better nutrients. They benefit from good hydration, just as we do. Bacteria are full of water just as we are. In short, the efficiency of your whole inner ecology rises when hydration and nutrition are partnered and absorbed together. This just makes intuitive sense.

Fermenting as a Form of Filtering?

Pilgrims crossing Spain's deserts in the twelfth century recovered by nightly drinking mead, also known as honey wine, a fermented beverage that both cleansed contaminated water and helped their immune system. Probiotics in fermented drinks indisputably bind toxins, molds, and heavy metals and carry them out of the body without getting absorbed.[3] In effect, ingesting fermented foods and drink helps our bodies function far better than our water filters.

You may have heard how important the microbiome is to providing health for your gut; indeed, that is where most of our bacteria live. Our bacteria are what help keep unabsorbed and too-large food particles from leaking back into your bloodstream. The gut microbiota have a role in the development of the gut lining. They increase the density of small intestinal capillaries and, in so doing, influence gut physiology and gut motility. We now know the gut microbiome is involved in digestion, immune stimulation, and metabolism of the host (that's you).[4]

To understand the microbiome, think of your body as an aquarium, full of lots of little floating things that need well-circulating water that is highly oxygenated, negatively charged, and full of wonderful nutrients.

SEASONAL MICROBES

As much as our bodies react to seasons, microbes, too, have seasonal patterns. Each season of fresh food brings its own kind of microbes, and the closer we eat to the seasons around us, the more our natural environment can support us to thrive in our unnatural, indoor environments. Dr. Lara Hooper runs one of the foremost microbiome research labs at University of Texas Southwestern Medical Center. She has revealed another major discovery: Microbacteria also function on circadian rhythms... they sleep too! They need us to be outdoors so they know whether it is night or day. Even inside us, down in that dark, they can read the angle of light waves and know what time it is and what season it is. Slowly we are putting together what our indoor life has cost our whole inner system. Seasonal eating has even more value than we realized, and a recent Stanford University study shows how that is true. They reviewed the habits of the Hadza, a nomadic tribe in Tanzania, still practicing ancient strategies of food consumption. Hadza survive and flourish by shifting through the seasons to different landscapes and therefore different foods. They eat what is seasonably available, and not only does that strategy provide a broader spectrum of nutrients but a broader spectrum of good bacteria. Because they have more diversity in their microbiome, their immunity and resilience to illness is also heightened, precisely because of their seasonal eating practice. Added to that, the very food they eat assists in their digestion and absorption of these new and diverse microbes. The bacteria are matched to the foods that are more available. Samuel Smits, the lead author of the study, found that there were striking differences, with some microbes disappearing and reappearing during different seasons.[5]

Dr. John Douillard, DC, who is a widely respected expert on nutrition and a leading Ayurvedic expert, confirms that our gut microbes are meant to change seasonally. There is a reason Dr. Douillard is so excited about this aforementioned Stanford study. He has long been a proponent of seasonal eating. As author of *The 3-Season Diet*, he has developed a modern three-season plan for food shopping in everyday grocery stores. Our Quench Plan, by offering seasonal food choices, maximizes nutrient contents from foods. Local eating, as much as possible, delivers these newfound benefits. As soon as fruit is plucked, it starts to lose its nutrient content. This is not even mentioning the waste and cost it takes to get the fruit thousands of miles away. We draw from Dr. Douillard's important work on seasonal eating by providing smoothies for hot and cold weather changes. He goes on to say, "When we do not eat seasonally, our microbiome is quickly disconnected to the intelligence of nature, and much of our genetic dependence on seasonal microbes is lost."

THE BENEFITS OF SMOOTHIES AND JUICES

In our Quench Plan, we recommend smoothies over juicing. We are not against juicing, as juice does carry gel water from inside the plants and is still a better, more nutritious way to hydrate in many situations than a bottle of water alone. Nonetheless, Quench is about *optimal* hydration. Juicing extracts the juice and filters out the pulp, and smoothies blend in the whole vegetable or fruit, retaining the fiber. Smoothies allow the full food benefits of plant material to remain in the drink. The sponging effect of plant fibers creates long-lasting, slow-release absorption of water and is therefore the best possible strategy for staying moist and youthful inside.

DR. DANA'S CASE STUDY

Evelyn

Evelyn is a thirty-nine-year-old who is healthy on pretty much all fronts: She takes relatively good care of herself, watches her diet, and has no significant past medical history nor takes any medication outside of supplements.

But despite all this, she had unexplained pain behind her right knee, and it had been bothering her for about a year. (Note: Don't wait a year with pain to see a doctor!) It worsened when she sat for long periods, so much so that when she would stand to "walk it out" after being sedentary for a period of time, she anticipated the pain—to the point where she actually became *more* sedentary over time. Her exercise consisted mostly of walking and a Pilates class once a week, which sometimes made the pain worse the next day.

After a physical exam and blood work, we went over her diet. I asked her if she thought she drank enough water. She said probably not, which is the same answer most of my patients give. I sent her home with the Quench program, consisting of one smoothie a day, micromovements, and a morning glass of water with lemon and sea salt.

We had a follow-up after two weeks, and I asked how she was feeling. She said she felt fine. When I asked about her pain, she was astonished to realize that it was gone. She'd actually forgotten about it! At another follow-up about six months later, she told me the pain had never come back—and to top it off, she was ten pounds lighter. She has been pain-free ever since.

The plant fibers, or cellulose, in essence sweep clean the microsized toxins, cellular waste, and debris that are constantly coming in from our industrial environments. Plant compounds can even buffer us from electromagnetic assaults, which can create mineral imbalances.[6] With smoothies there is no tossing out the precious pulp. The many synergistic plant compounds and biological cofactors hidden in that pulp material is not lost or wasted. We still have not yet identified all that is available in a Mother Nature package. Smoothies get us that all-important fiber missing from typical diets. Those plant fibers create the optimal environment for our microbiome and all the good bacteria, which need hydration, too! Smoothies fill us up beautifully and run our systems efficiently with less cost than juicing. They feed and nourish us and our microbiome, and therefore they diminish cravings and the weight that comes with those insatiable yearnings. Quench them with smoothies!

Smoothies provide:

- Absorption of hydration
- Time-released hydration
- Dense nutrients
- Dense fiber
- Food for us
- Food for our microbiome
- Microcleansing
- Buffering from environmental and electromagnetic toxins
- No waste
- Cost-effective nutrition
- Diminished cravings

Juicing provides:

- Nutritious hydration
- Easily absorbed minerals and vitamins
- Immediate bioavailability
- But watch out for higher sugar absorption.

The Million-Year-Old Diet

The Hadza of Northern Tanzania are one of the communities Gina studied for her original anthropological research on how desert- or dry-environment groups survive on so little water. The Hadza live in a mostly arid savannah region, and though they have contact with other cultures, most Hadza choose to continue their ancestral way of life.

Professor Tim Spector, from the Genetic Epidemiology department at King's College London, spent three days with the Hadzas, eating only what they ate. Indeed, the diet matches Gina's records from her original research; Spector recorded drinking a morning "smoothie" that provided a high level of hydration and nutrition. His account of his diet was fascinating.[7]

He spoke of the baobab fruit as a staple in the Hadza diet. The fruit, packed with vitamins, fat, and fiber, has a hard coconut-like shell with chalky flesh inside that surrounds a seed. Spector described how the Hadza blended the chalky substance with water until it had a thick, milky consistency. This, for them, was a typical breakfast. He also described eating wild berries called Kongorobi berries, which have twenty times the fiber and polyphenols compared with the berries we get in the grocery store today. A late lunch consisted of a few high-fiber tubers.

In his account, Spector records in extraordinary detail a diet that functionally matches our Quench Plan, starting with smoothies in the morning. High fiber and fats, stirred in with water, creates long-lasting hydration in dry conditions and are satiating as well. With the current popularity of diets mimicking our ancestors, such as Paleo diets, one important feature is not commonly known: Like the Hadza, ancient peoples ate a great deal of plants. Far more than meats. These high-plant diets served to supplement their hydration, a strategy especially used in arid environments.

Spector goes on to say that the Hadza eat a large diversity of plants and animals yet spend little time hunting and gathering. Makes you wonder which is the more advanced society: Hunter-gatherer societies that work fewer hours a day to feed their family, or our modern one that works eight-plus hours a day.[8]

Seasonal eating offers a lot of cues to our inner mechanisms about how to run efficiently through the year. We may not know yet what these relationships are, but if we eat seasonally and get outdoors often, we may not have to know everything about environmental symbiosis to reap the benefits.

FERVENT FERMENTATION

You have probably heard about fermented foods lately—and for good reason. Foods that basically sit around and "age" gain properties that amplify the nutritional value of food. Fermentation is the most ancient process for enhancing and preserving food. Fermented foods have been through a process in which natural bacteria feed on sugars and carbs, creating lactic acid. This process also creates beneficial bacteria and enzymes and helps assemble omega-3 fatty acids, and in turn helps your digestive tract do its job.

Yet today, we diminish our natural bacteria with antibiotics, sterilization, and overkill. Fermenting foods is a very, very ancient strategy, found in all cultures, to provide preserved and highly supportive nutrients to this bacteria. Fermented foods were the original preservatives. Fermentation made refrigerators unnecessary. We co-evolved with these bacteria and they ignite many functions to run our systems well. Let's get them back into our daily diets. Bacteria are lightning quick at adapting, and they quickly figure out the best way to support us, because in supporting us they support themselves. Great houseguests!

Are plants drugs?

Did you know that the word *drug* is derived from the French *drogue*, which means "dried herb"? The word's origin strongly suggests that the earliest drugs were taken from plants, much like they are today. It may surprise you, though, that they still account for approximately 40 percent of pharmaceuticals sold in the United States. Just looking at the amount of money made in that industry, you would think they were on to something. And they are: Plants do the body good, and we are just finding out just how much.

Not all our smoothie recipes have fermented ingredients, but we share tricks that you can use just as you need or want. And remember that fiber in our smoothies is food for your microbiome—these fibers are sometimes known as prebiotics. Now you don't have to ask why you would want to drink a smoothie with fermented materials in it. It's surprising how delicious they can be.

Our Quench strategy, both old and new, helps us conserve and protect water on Earth. Water extracted from our foods, from plants, rather than drained from aquifers, means we use water to nurture plants. We let the plants transform that water and in return gain a better quality water from the plants we eat. Eat your water, indeed.

CHAPTER 3

Move That Water

Fascia and Hydration

If there is magic on this planet, it is contained in water.

—*Loren Eiseley*

How does water actually get into you where it's needed, to moisten your skin and saturate your brain, muscles, organs, and tissues? We have a brand-new and beautiful answer to these questions. It is called fascia, pronounced "FASH-ah."

Fascia, in the shortest possible definition, equals tissue. It is a specialized, extraordinarily gossamer, gauzy tissue that lies not only under your skin, but also between and around your organs and bones. And there are miles of it. In fact, we are shot through and through with fascia. It is one of the deepest anatomical mysteries that scientists are currently exploring. This mysterious territory is as exciting now as when the first human body was examined. Dr. James Oschman, an American biophysicist who had a four-year stint at Cambridge University to research fluid and electrical transport in cells, says it best: "Fascia forms the largest system in the body, as it is the system that touches all the other systems."[1] And as we're learning, fascia's function is key to the work of hydration. You may never have heard of fascia unless you have had a bout of plantar fasciitis, a common but painful inflammation of the connective tissue in the arch of your foot. Movements that stretch this fascia bring hydration back into this tissue and speed recovery.

Yet until recently, fascia was seen as a merely protective wrapping to keep organs and muscles in place, much like Saran Wrap. Dissectionists would peel and toss it away, as you do plastic wrap, to get to the important stuff: organs and the skeletal, vascular, muscular, and nerve systems. That tossed-away, plasticlike wrap was already desiccated and dehydrated by the time a student dissectionist got to it. It did not look important. It wasn't until 2005 that scientists saw fascia for the first time, fully alive and fully hydrated. This stunning video went viral immediately.

DR. DANA'S CASE STUDY

Jeffrey

A physiatrist in my practice recommended that I see thirty-year-old Jeffrey. He had been treating him for his foot issues, particularly very painful plantar fasciitis. Jeffrey was given exercises and had orthotics made for his shoes, but two months later there was minimal improvement in his foot pain. He was very overweight, and my colleague thought that might be the reason.

When Jeffrey came in, we talked about his history.

"I have always been overweight—even when I was a child. I have gotten as heavy as 330, but I am down to 250, mostly by cutting out carbs. But it has been few months and I haven't lost any more weight. I wish I could work out more, but my foot…"

As we continued, he told me he had fainted twice from dehydration in the past. I did bloodwork on him, and while we waited for test results to return, I asked him to start the Quench program. He was a little hesitant, since he was so used to thinking the only thing that worked for him was a very-low-carb diet; he was afraid of eating fruits, and even some vegetables, because of their carbohydrate content. I assured him it wouldn't hurt him—that there were *good* carbs—and I went over a healthy eating plan similar to what we recommend in this book.

When we met for a follow-up two weeks later, he was six pounds lighter and was exercising more, because his foot was feeling better. Six months later, he is down to 218, exercising regularly, eating a whole-foods diet and following the Quench rules religiously. His plantar fasciitis is history. His day includes a big glass of water and sea salt right after waking up, a glass of water just before every meal, and usually two smoothies a day.

That was the year Dr. Jean-Claude Guimberteau, a brilliant French surgeon and expert in hand reconstruction, performed a quite delicate operation. To better see the tissues during surgery, he stuck a fiber-optic camera under the skin of the patient. Normally, red blood would have obscured the complicated underlay of fascia, but this time he clamped off the blood vessels so he could better see the fascia tissue. The fiber-optic camera recorded and exposed an exquisite mesh that was pulsing and moving—almost as if it were breathing. And this clear netting was *transporting water droplets*, revealing for the first time that fascia is one of the body's major water transport system.[2] This video revealed the expanding, contracting irrigation system as it passed water along its tubing. We could finally see fascia watering our tissues, just as if it were irrigating a garden.

Along with gel water, fascia detection should be considered among the top discoveries of our time. This eureka moment immediately altered our view of how our bodies retain hydration and move it throughout our bodies. The camera clearly revealed that fascia has hollow tubing and slide-like sheets that actually send the water that you drink into your tissues. We include a link to the video in our Resources if you'd like to view it and see for yourself.[3]

This discovery proves that fascia plays a vital role connecting hydration with body movement. Any motion—turning, stretching, twisting—activates this water-delivery system. Fascia works its hydraulic pumping action by constriction and release. It literally works as a hydraulic pump! The very word *hydraulic* means "movement by water."

This is truly a magnificent revelation. Fascia, instead of merely filler tissue, a casing system for our body parts, is a distinct, functional newfound hydraulic system in its own right. A transparent, almost invisible mobile system, fascia is, therefore, key to water transport. We can now trace how water gets to our tissues and cells. In fact, movement is the necessary next step in hydration, after drinking. Movement actually draws hydration all the way through our tissues into our cells.[4] It is quite literally the other half of hydration. Drinking starts the hydration process, but movement completes it.

ALL FASCIA DOES

Fascia has near miraculous multiple functions. Yes, its webbing holds your muscles to your bones and rests your eyes in their sockets. Yet, this extraordinary new view of fascia as the body's irrigation system holds another surprise. Fascia not only transports water, it is actually made up of water—gel water, plus collagen—the most abundant protein in the body. Together they form the body's flexible, malleable scaffolding. Let's get a handle on these new discoveries. What is fascia actually doing?

Fascia is an electrical system, run on and made of water. Traditionally, the nervous system was thought to be the only electrical transmitter in the body, but now we realize that fascia is also transmitting additional electrical charges. How is it even possible that a crucial electrical system in the body is only now being recognized and charted? Water conducts electricity, so it makes sense that fascia, made of water, would as well. In fact, we now know that fascia conducts electricity at exponentially faster rates. Though there are forty-seven miles of nerves in the average human body, there are far more miles of fascia. Fascia surrounds every organ and vessel we have, and that includes nerves. And because of its speed of conduction, fascia is rather like the fiber-optic system of communication and information of the body.

Dr. Mae-Wan Ho, a biophysicist and nanoparticle scientist who founded the Institute for Science and Society in London, pointed out that nanotubes, which exist inside fascia's microscopic water crystals, are aligned by collagen fibers. This combination, she posits, fulfills all the criteria for superconduction. Her take is that, though we don't know the exact mechanism for how the gel water creates electricity superconducting is occurring inside each of us all the time.[5] This accelerated information service, to and from our cells, charges itself through simple movement. Wow, could we get this system for our cell phones?

Fascia is also a sonic system, one that utilizes vibrational energy and sound energy. This opens up a world of diagnostic and therapeutic possibilities of healing and vitality. Doctors are already using ultrasound therapy for tendon pain. Healthy, well-hydrated fascia responds to vibration. Dr. Sungchul Ji, from Rutgers University, has a brilliantly simple analogy for understanding how water molecules could become more efficient. He posits that gel water, with its unique crystalline alignment, acts like a tuning fork. All the vibrational waves sync and become coherent, laser-like, and less scattered. They move together, creating a new and changed resonance.

Even Albert Einstein insisted, "Everything in life is vibration," so why wouldn't water be? This vibrational sync or coherence creates more efficient function. It is possible it can organize and amplify electrical charge, "because of the extreme sensitivity of water molecules to sound vibration and their molecular environment changes," Ji says.[6]

To spread the new interest on fascia into public awareness, it took, and takes, many researchers in many disciplines. Holistic health practitioners, dancers, and massage therapists knew from their experiences that something was going on with fascia that had yet to be defined. Even now, the field of fascial research is like the proverbial story of the blind men describing an elephant; each describes only a part of the elephant. And like the elephant, fascia is comically complex.

Fascia still remains full of unknowns, but one thing is certain: It requires hydration to do its many jobs. While fascia research is fairly new and revolutionary, techniques for manipulating fascia and keeping it elastic are ancient. Yoga, tai chi and qi gong, and, of course, dancing are only some of the widespread practices that produce flexible centenarians.

To experience fascia at work, try this: Put your arm straight out, elbow stiff, with palm up, fingers splayed as wide as you can.

Start with your palm facing up and then gently, as far around as possible, rotate. Try to draw a complete circle in the air with your thumb. Now, check in with yourself to see how far the rotation went. It's possible to feel the twist all the way from your fingertips up to the shoulder blade in your back. Far more of your fascia is at work in this stretch than your muscles, tendons, and nerves. We hope you can notice that when you stick your thumb far out, you get more of a whole-body stretch.

Another way to become aware of your fascial system is to check with your spine throughout the day. Are you sitting up, or are you hunched over? Fix your posture, which uses more fascia than spine to hold you up. The more often you do it, the more you improve flow. And you'll look better, too! Hydration and vitality are also tied to longevity. Here's why: When hunched over, you are constricting your tissues and your breathing, and so further restricting that flow of water in your body. We don't want to treat our spine like a folded, squeezed, or constricted hose, blocking the flow of water and interfering with our breathing capacity. Breathing is another unsung source of hydration. Breathing pulls vapor out of the air. Hunching over squeezes the intestinal tract, which again kinks digestive function and its *flow*. Posture affects each of these bodily functions. This flow, remember, is not only hydraulic in nature but also electrical, because *water flow is electrical flow.* Water is all about movement. Indeed, if it isn't moving, it isn't living, and neither are we. This may help you think about exercise and movement differently, knowing that you can have a greater impact on your health and well-being by doing frequent gentle stretches than by marathon sessions of crunches and presses.

Stretching yourself out and unkinking here and there throughout your day now makes a lot of sense.

FASCIA AND SPORTS

Modern sports medicine has also developed techniques for restoring fascia to health. It is in the world of high-performance athletics that we glean much practical information about fascia and how to treat injury. Soccer's top sports physiotherapist, Klaus Eder, works with damaged fascia. He noticed, via specialized ultrasound, that a film of gel flows between fascial layers. So he carefully and slowly separates layers matted together through injury, thus enabling the gel layer to return between the tissues. The gel layer enables tissues to again slide freely, allowing athletes to return to the field more quickly. Eder, to help us understand fascia from his perspective, has described injured fascia as a sweater that has been washed in too-hot water, losing its elasticity. When fascia is matted or toughened, this can make it more prone to injury and reduces the access of nutrition, blood, and oxygen to the area. Hydration is your first intervention with a sports injury. In addition to reaching for an ice pack, you should reach for a glass.

FASCIA IS SUSPENSION ARCHITECTURE

Every fibrous strand of muscle is encased in a filmy sheath of buffering fascia, like an elastic wrapping, but beyond that, fascia has a biomechanical support life of its own. Thomas Myers, a pioneer in myo (muscle) fascial connection, has a wonderful word for this: *tensegrity*.[7] This word was originally coined by the legendary architect and engineer Buckminster Fuller. Fuller used *tensegrity* in reference to the strength of building structures using balanced cables. Myers applies this concept to the body by comparing fascia to cables on bridges. "In the normal healthy state, the fascia is relaxed and wavy in configuration. It has the ability to stretch and move without restriction. When one experiences physical trauma, emotional trauma, scarring, or inflammation, however, the fascia loses its pliability. It becomes tight, restricted, and a source of tension to the rest of the body."[8] He further explains that anything from a major trauma, such as a car accident or surgery, to smaller infractions like poor posture or repetitive overuse can have cumulative effects on the body, and in particular the fascial system. The changes trauma causes in the fascial system influence the comfort and function of our body. When an injury or trauma occurs, it can impose restrictions on the fascia that affect our range of motion, flexibility, and stability and can cause a myriad of symptoms such as pain and headaches. Hydration should be the first step in repairing our fascia along with physical therapy and other modalities. Hydration returns fascia's elasticity.

FASCIA IS ALERT

Another dazzling discovery, by German pioneer Dr. Robert Schleip, has shown that fascia is populated with receptors and nerve endings.[9] This is where spatial receptors in the body are most densely packed. These sensors or receptors fire *when the tissue stretches* and in this way allow our brain and body to register where our body is in space. Fascia and the autonomic nervous system appear to be intimately connected. Our sense of proprioception, that inner GPS, is what keeps us three-dimensional beings adjusted in space. Now imagine that our spatial awareness depends on the level of hydration.

That clumsy fall you had? Muscles are the last ones to get the news. The receptor system of the fascia is the first point of awareness. Dehydration in this sensitive system diminishes our space perception and balance, which is why properly hydrated fascia is key for younger people seeking optimum sports performance, as well as older people who want to avoid a nasty fall.

Here's an example of the fascial system at work: to train spatial awareness in young kids who lack it, occupational therapists put close-fitting vests on them. The kids can then sense where their bodies are. We can now understand how that works: The therapists are further stimulating receptor firing in the fascia through the touch and pressure of the fabric vest.

This vest therapy recalls another touch-stimulating therapy. Dry brushing is mostly known for its exfoliating effects, which enhances blood circulation throughout the skin and lymphatic drainage. Dry brushing certainly does that, but in addition it can especially help fascia in three distinct ways. Think about what dry brushing is doing under the skin. It stimulates all those different kinds of receptors and nerve endings; it provides pinpoint compression from the bristles, not unlike a superficial acupuncture treatment; and when you drag a dry brush across dry skin, the brushing pushes fluid across the fascial network. A three-for-one benefit.

Brush up?

You can get a natural bristle dry body brush at any drugstore or natural health food store. They are usually labeled for dry body brushing. To practice dry brushing, use long strokes up the limbs, which draws fluid toward the lymph collection nodes in your groin area and armpits. Then brush across the buttocks, torso, and back, always brushing upward toward your heart. As you bend over and stretch to reach these areas, you are also doing a beneficial fascial stretch.

Another version of dry brushing is simple self-massage. We will share some self-massage techniques from ancient India and China in chapter 7.

FASCIA AND ACUPUNCTURE

Acupuncture has long been associated with pain management. These new discoveries in fascia corroborate the theories behind the ancient practice. Recent research has documented that neuroreceptors are not equally distributed in the fascia but occur in concentrated canals or channels. Helene Langevin, a neurologist at the University of Vermont, sees an 80 percent overlap of fascial concentration points with ancient maps that illustrate the meridian lines for acupuncture. These overlap areas are thickly populated with those firing receptors and nerve endings. Even more amazing, her team was able to capture on film fascia reacting to acupuncture needle insertions. They were witness to a remarkable sight: Fascia reacts to needle insertion by collecting thickly around the needle tip, in effect making a stronger weave or density of collagen fibers.[10] Do we know what this means yet? No. We speculate this is how acupuncture helps with pain. It's a whole new world, but it may be that research is unveiling a better understanding of the effective practices of Eastern medicine.

FASCIA IS TRULY FASCIA-NATING

Fascia still remains full of unknowns, but one thing is certain: It requires hydration to do its job. While fascia research is fairly new, techniques for manipulating fascia and keeping it elastic are ancient. Yoga, tai chi and qi gong, and, of course, dancing, are some of the popular practices that produce flexibility as well as longevity.

Will you feel differently discovering that you're full of fascia? We hope so, and we will show you how to activate your fascia yourself. We have experienced our own bodies differently even while researching and writing about fascia. For one, we no longer let ourselves sit for long sessions at the computer without many intervals of small movements and stretching. We became more aware of the living fascial system inside us that we could enliven simply by giving it our attention and by giving our body short breaks. Let's call them charge breaks. Our fascia and body reward us in turn with a fluid vibrancy and more energy. How exciting to discover a new irrigation system hiding inside us.

CHAPTER 4

How Motion Keeps You Hydrated

The Science of Micromovements

Water is the driving force of all nature.

—*Leonardo da Vinci*

The big surprise we want to share is that *motion keeps you hydrated*. You might think that exercise would dehydrate you, and it can, but movement is necessary for proper hydration. We already know of hundreds of studies that prove just how important exercise and movement is to our health. That is nothing new. But our groundbreaking news is that movement plays a critical role that's even more fundamental. Movement moves hydration down to the cellular level. And we are finding it doesn't take a lot of movement at all; the simplest and smallest motion can help get water to all parts of your body. Movement is the second half of the hydration formula. Without movement, hydration doesn't get all the way to our fascia and ultimately to our cells.

In 2016, a major study was published involving 12,776 British women who were followed closely to identify one thing and one thing only: Would fidgeting protect their longevity?[1] It did. Women who didn't fidget much and who sat for seven hours a day or more, were associated with a whopping 43 percent *increase* in their risk for *all-cause mortality*. Compare that to women who fell into middle or even high categories of fidgeting. They had no greater risk of dying even when *they sat for more than seven hours a day*. It all goes to show that motion leads to health—even small motions. Even if you're seated. Even if it's a fidget.

Another quirky study brings this news into total clarity. As reported in the *American Journal of Physiology* in 2016,[2] eleven young men were asked to sit still for three hours and fidget just one leg. What lengths we go to for research! But they found some very disconcerting results. One minute of fidgeting every four minutes *improved* the circulation of the fidget leg, but the vascular *rigidity* of the nonfidget leg actually increased from the baseline measurement. The authors concluded that the "simple behavior of fidgeting is sufficient to counteract the detrimental effects of prolonged sitting." Thus they provided original evidence that the negative impact of immobility for extended periods can be avoided with small amounts of movement.

CELLS AS MOTION DETECTORS

In this chapter, the most important takeaway is that motion ignites cell function. Your cells are literally motion detectors. You are your own engine, designed to ignite yourself through motion. Any kind of motion. Unless you are moving, your cells are not in high function. They are not hydrated or charged. The *kind* of movement is important—we're not talking about running a marathon or going to the gym for hours on end. The simplest, smallest motion can help draw water and electrical charge to all parts of your body. With *Quench* we'll show you how easy they are.

How does this all work, movement and hydration? It comes back to our amazing network beneath the skin, the fascia. As you move, the pulleylike action of muscle, fascia, and skin, stretching across your skeletal architecture, simultaneously pushes hydration more deeply into your tissues and squeezes your body's cells into action.

Any motion, large or small—a tilt of the head, a slight shoulder raise, or a large stride—stretches tissues and generates electricity. This is a principle happening all over nature, relying on straightforward mechanical stress, and the scientific name for this process is piezoelectricity (peez-o-electricity), or "pressure electricity." Piezoelectrical movement helps hydration seep into your tissues and charge your cells. The movements don't have to be big or enduring. Cells are tiny, and tiny motion is a big movement to a cell.

Pierre and Jacques Curie identified the piezoelectric effect in 1880, showing mechanical stress can be converted into voltage. Today, researchers have identified that this same principle is active all the way through to the cellular and molecular level. Yale University's researchers show in the journal *Cellular Neuroscience, Neurodegeneration and Repair* that piezoelectric proteins already exist within the cell. These proteins are responsible for sensing motion and stretch, and those small motions activate many functions in the cell.[3]

> ### Squeezing Makes Energy
>
> Did you know that just squeezing a quartz crystal between your fingers creates electricity? This is not so different from how computer touch screens work, because they are made from liquid crystals. Liquid crystalline structure, the exact kind found in gel water, responds to pressure.

INTRODUCING MICROMOVEMENTS

If you are moving every day in the same old ways, the same habits, likely half of you is underactivated. We are actually three-dimensional creatures. In fact, new pathways of movement stretch our fascia and get those cells out of the sluggish, compressed life of sitting all the time. We often think that keeping a painful muscle still is the best way to heal it. It's a protective instinct, but using tiny, gentle movements to stretch sore body parts can actually accelerate healing.

Do you feel sluggish? If you suffer from low energy, it's likely not your fault. It is not a character defect. You're not lazy. Rather, we are conditioned by our contemporary culture not to move— and it's costing all of us our vitality. It starts at childhood, when we're put behind desks at school, and it continues into adulthood, when most of us are tethered to a computer, a chair, and a car for eight or more hours per day. If you're not moving, you're not energizing yourself. It's not your fault you aren't moving as much as nature intended. But perhaps you can discover just how much life and energy is still in you. Perhaps there's a way to put a little bit of movement back in your day, to fully hydrate your cells and bring some energy back to your day, no matter where you work or what your age.

You don't have to get up and run a marathon to activate your cells. You can use micromovements. Notice we are not using the word *exercise* here but *movement*, and for a reason. Movement and the energy it ignites may well get you further down the line to the ultimate goal of regular exercise. But that is not the focus here. And if you are already an exercise buff, it is still important to keep your body flexible with 360-degree micromovements. Our focus here is on the new knowledge that the energy micromovements bring our cells comes from the delivery of hydration.

Throughout your day you can keep your system from going to "sleep" just like your computers do when they sit around unused. Micromovements are the answer to efficiently keeping your cells, and your body, "on" to the end of the day.

LITTLE MOVES LEAD TO BIG MOVES

We are not against exercise. Our purpose in this chapter is to connect even the smallest movement with cell activation, based on hydration's capacity to delivery energy. There are plenty of books written about the physical and psychological benefits of exercise—some of which we mention in the Resources section. For those who can't or don't exercise, these small micromovements can be the impetus to get you exercising more formally. You only need a little movement to accomplish a lot...Just as the name indicates, micromovements are small motions tailored to help our bodies work better—even random fidgeting counts. But our precise micromovements will get you even more energy.

FULL BODY FLOW: IN AND OUT

In *Quench*, we provide a strategic set of small, targeted movements to purposefully move your body top to toe. We devised our micromovements based on these newly revealed discoveries about fidgeting, which confirm the power of tiny movement. But *Quench* gets you further with three-dimensional awareness, front and back, so unused tissue doesn't go stiff, dormant, or to sleep like your computer. We are meant to rotate, looking behind us often, rolling our shoulders, ankles, hips, and, yes, eyes, to further draw in hydration. Once you have the micromovement concept, you want to find stiff places in your body and get some small movements targeted there. You will naturally start devising your own custom micromovements. Once you understand you can move anywhere, in your bed, in your chair, in your car, in line, with small unobtrusive micromovements and see how you instantly feel better, you will love micromovements.

In addition, these microvements aid in the outflow work of expelling old fluids full of cellular waste. Limited mobility starts with underuse, which accumulates cellular waste and creates inflammation. You want that 360-degree, full range of motion, so every tissue in your body has in-and-out flow to remain supple and healthy.

We have up to now been focused on the concept of drawing hydration into our cells. Now we want to focus on the power of water to draw waste *out* of our cells, indeed, out of all our tissues. True hydration isn't just *in* but also *out*. The entire lymphatic flow system, our inner sanitation department, is utterly dependent on our own movement to work. If you are not using many small movements throughout the day, you're accumulating waste. Your system is backing up with sludge and looking to you to get moving. If you aren't engaged in this natural process, the waste material will slowly begin to inflame your tissues, interfere with efficient function, and make you old before your time. To that end, we offer a special strategy: twisting. We will provide at the end of the chapter a full-body guide for these on-the-go micromovements.

LET'S TWIST AGAIN

The twisting motion—whether your arms, legs, neck, or spine—induces a superefficient technique for waste management. Think of twisting as if you were wringing out a wet dishcloth, getting old wastewater out. Twisting or spiraling, so often found in classic tai chi, yoga, and even other forms of practice like simple dancing, will rotate your spine and give it a fabulous spiral squeeze. And once you release from the twist, you then draw up fresh fluids, full of oxygen and nutrients. Twisting is, in effect, an efficient anti-inflammatory tactic.

MICROMOVEMENT THROUGH YOUR DAY

You can intercept those times of day where you feel fatigue. For example, while you are on your cell phone, stretch your chin over your shoulder a couple of times, or maybe do some ankle circles. Unlike aerobic exercise, where the typical motto is "No pain, no gain," twisting micromovements can provide a lot of effect for very little effort. Remember those fidget studies?

It's inspiring to discover we can do micromovement anywhere, anytime. How often do you look over your shoulder, except maybe to back the car out of the driveway? Try it now; go slow and do what's comfortable, but really try to get your chin aligned with your shoulder—and notice how that simple movement activates whole muscle groups in your back. Muscles that you don't usually use in your daily grind. Use moments like being in your car or on your phone to do micromovements—it will help you break out of poor habitual positions that over time make us stiff, inflexible, and less mobile.

If you have perpetual neck and shoulder tension (and really, why wouldn't you, when you're tipped over screens and keyboards constantly?), these simple moves will restore you. Think of it as a physical therapy session, not at a therapist's office but throughout the day. This affects all of us who are texting on our phones 24/7.

Daily motion is the very first thing on the list of nine identified practices in the "Blue Zones," those hot spots of longevity around the globe. The elders in these blue zones hike and hoe and haul and garden right alongside their family members of all ages. We long to end up as this kind of aged person, independent, alert, fluid, humorous about life, and still able to care for others. Could we end it any better? Your body is still full of endless moves you've never tried before, and your cells are eager responders whenever you give them a little pump, push, or squeeze. Who knew that hydration, and hydration transferred into our cells through motion, could get us to this level of lively longevity? Water has always been and will always be the fountain of youth.

ALIGNING MICROMOVEMENTS WITH MICROMEMORY

Norman Doidge, MD, a neurologist and the author of the groundbreaking book *The Brain That Changes Itself*,[4] shows that when neurons fire together, as when movement and memory are activated at the same time, they make stronger connections.

So, ask yourself: When was the last time you felt *really* good? Healthy, vibrant? Full of energy? Under what conditions? Can you identify or recall if it was during a time you were more active? Hold that image and see if you can reactivate that body memory going forward even with small movements through your day. Use our supersimple micromovements, ones that anyone can do, and couple them with the memory of your happy motion moments. This combination, fidgeting to a happy memory, is a winning one, firing and aligning brain cells to body movement. And have you heard of the tapping solution?[5] Not tap dancing, but tapping lightly on key spots on the face, head, and body with positive affirmations for pain and trauma relief? Veterans use it with an accelerated recovery rate from posttraumatic stress disorder, often in under ten sessions. A 69 percent recovery rate was documented, higher than any medical intervention.[6]

DR. DANA'S CASE STUDY

Patricia

Patricia, a fifty-three-year-old magazine editor, flies every so often for work. Recently, after getting off a flight from London, she noticed swelling in her feet. Her shoes were tight, and her ankles and calves felt heavy—it was an uncomfortable feeling. She came to see me for relief. I reassured her that it wasn't anything serious, but she did have a case of edema, a buildup of excess fluid in the body's tissues. A big cause of edema can be dehydration—and as you have read, flying can a big trigger for dehydration. (See the Why Do I Get So Thirsty When I Fly? section in the Introduction for tips on flying and hydration.)

I gave Patricia a few tips on hydrating and prescribed a few simple movements that would help with the swelling, including classic pelvic tilts. Patricia saw immediate results: She e-mailed me a few days later, remarking, "I can't believe it! I can see my ankles again!"

She marveled at how quickly the swelling went down after doing the movement techniques each day.

Here's the pelvic tilt movement that helps move circulation through your lower extremities: Lay on your back, knees bent with feet flat on the floor. Palms on the floor, too, and lift and lower your hips. Do three sets of five tilts. Pelvic tilts can be done in bed, too, and can be added to your morning micromovements.

Moving the Years and Illness Away

Sanford Bennett, known as "the man who turned young at seventy," had become determined to turn his life around after suffering chronic illnesses that left him practically bedridden. By his fifties, he had recovered completely and published a book in 1907 entitled *Exercising in Bed* that chronicled his transformation and inspired some of our micromovements. Bennett, convinced that he aged prematurely by the accumulation of waste material in his tissues, thought if he twisted, constricted, and relaxed his muscles he could move waste out through his blood system. Bennett may have been hazy on the particulars, but he wasn't wrong on principles, and his body was proof. By age seventy, he was visibly a much younger man. He's a great example of how twisting movement can be so beneficial, even in bed.

Joseph Pilates is another great pioneer in exercise. He grew up with numerous health issues, including rickets and asthma, and he took up exercise and strength building to battle his conditions. During World War I, after seeing soldiers who were too weak to get out of bed in an internment camp hospital, he devised a simple pulley system made from the bedsprings. He had them practice small targeted movements, convinced these movements were essential for boosting their physical health and their morale and mental acuity. Today, the Pilates method is just as likely to be used by toned suburban moms as by recovering battle veterans, but however they come to Pilates, it continues to help millions of fans stay fit. And in a beautiful irony, some forward-thinking hospitals use Pilates today, returning it to the site of origination.

THE THROUGHOUT-THE-DAY FULL-BODY MICROMOVEMENT MAP

Movement amplifies all the positive effects of hydration. Imagine yourself swinging out of bed without stiffness, fluid and free from pain. Picture yourself rising smoothly from your desk, easily lifting your child, or looking with ease over your shoulder as you back out your car. Hydration, along with the right moves, will help get you there. Later in the book we'll give you specific moves in the five-day Quench Plan that will change the very way you feel—slowing your aging trajectory and increasing your vitality—but here, our daily body map is designed to pick up where the five-day Quench Plan leaves off, for a lifetime of simple but comprehensive body movements.

DAILY BODY MOVEMENT MAP

We break down these exercises into two routines, the morning routine for the upper half of your body, and the afternoon one works the lower half of your body.

Morning Routine: Upper Body

Either standing or sitting, start with dropping your chin to your chest three times.

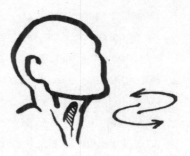

Feel the gentle tug across your shoulders and up your neck.

Draw some circles in the air with your chin, first small ones, eventually getting larger and looser

Draw a figure eight in air with your chin. Now try it with your nose. Alternate between chin and nose for an advanced perception experience.

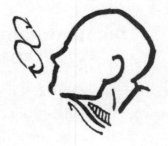

Move your ear to your shoulder a couple of times, as best as you are able, only to your comfort.

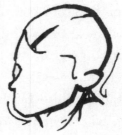

You don't need to actually have your ear touch your shoulder; you are just trying to activate all the muscles between them. Explore different positions, one or both shoulders up, shoulders down.

Swing your chin over your shoulder, look down, look up, and do it for your other shoulder.

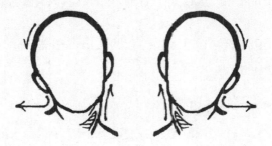

Move your elbows, with arms bent, backward as if you were trying to have them meet, until you feel your shoulder blades squeeze, two or three times.

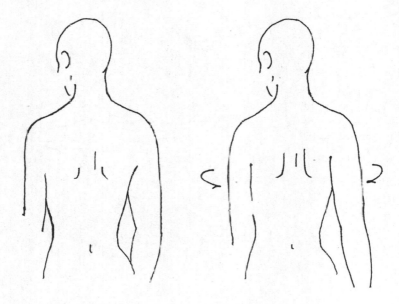

If you like, raise up your chin as you squeeze your elbows backward, but only to gentle comfort range.

Drop your chin to your chest, let out a breath, and then raise shoulders, scrunching them up to your ears. Quickly drop your shoulders.

First half of the body is done! Later this afternoon, work on the lower half of your body.

Afternoon Routine: Lower Body

Stand, or sit, with hips facing forward. Twist your torso to your right, trying to get your shoulders as perpendicular

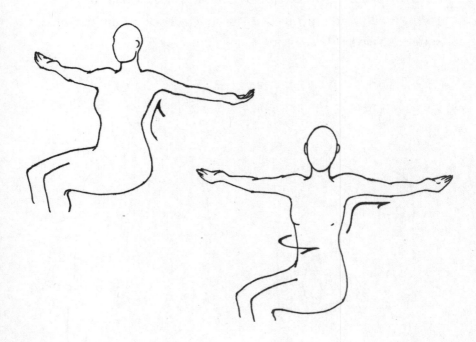

to your hips as long as it feels comfortable. You can press the edge of a desk or table for a little more push and even pulse it a little.

Now do the other side: Turn to your left, keeping your hips

facing forward, and try again to get
your shoulders to be perpendicular
to your hips, even grabbing the back
of your chair or a doorframe for a
gentle assist.

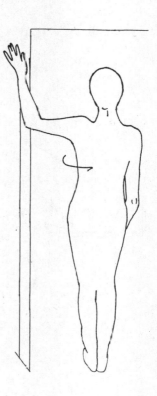

Stand in a doorway, and place
your raised hand above your head to
hold the doorframe. Twist forward
or backward until you can feel a pull
in your armpit. This is especially
good for women, moving waste out
of the breast area and improving
circulation.

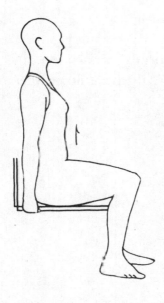

Sitting in a chair, drop your hands
to both sides of your chair, grab the
seat underneath, and pull up while
straightening your torso. Do this three
or four times.

While you are sitting, lift your knee
and roll your ankle in a circle. Don't
forget the other leg. Remember those
fidgeting studies.

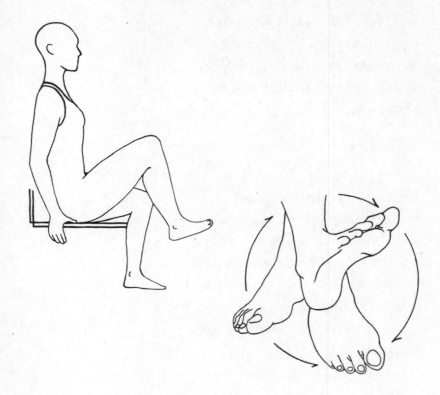

Wiggle your toes often.

Stand, and while your heels are firmly planted on the floor, raise your toes. Do one foot only, then the other, then both.

CHAPTER 5

Fat and Hydration

Oil and Water Do Mix

Formula for success: Rise early, work hard, strike oil.

—*J. Paul Getty*

Your health and youthfulness are directly linked to not only how much water you drink but also how well your body gets water into your cells. It is oils and fats that make cellular hydration possible. Water literally has to cross over an oil-guarded barrier to get inside your cell. You can drink all you want, but if water doesn't get past this membrane, hydration isn't really happening.

These cell membranes are made up primarily of fatty acids, called lipids, which help keep the membranes supple so that the cells can absorb water. New and important research documents that omega-3 fatty acids play especially key roles in keeping your cell membranes supple and your cells hydrated.[1] But that's not all. Omega-3s can also help increase the cell membrane surface area so that more water and nutrients can pass through.[2]

A diet loaded with damaging trans fats or fats damaged by heat leads to an accumulation of cholesterol and damaged fats right within the cell itself. This waste and toxic accumulation disrupts cellular communication[3] and impairs the uptake of nutrients and release of cellular wastes. This intracellular sludge over time impairs cellular functioning and will lead to an increase in cellular dehydration.

Cellular dehydration happens by accumulation of waste and toxins. As you get older, your cell membranes get stiff, and stiffened membranes block out not only hydration but also essential nutrients and oxygen from entering. These, of course, are the very things the cell needs in order to get waste products out. Accumulation and stiffness, it's a one-two punch. Fats to the rescue.

FAT: IT DOES YOUR BODY GOOD

Think of *fat* as a bad word? You're hardly alone. A recent survey from the International Food Information Council found that most Americans are confused about which kinds of fat are healthful. For years, many of us simply avoided *all* of them, thinking we were doing our hearts and waistlines a favor.[4] That's a mistake. While experts spent decades telling us that banishing fat would protect our hearts and keep us slim, now a wealth of research reveals the opposite. Most kinds of fat aren't just okay to eat. They're actually *essential* to your health.

Dietary fat—that is, fat you get from foods like avocados, olive oil, nuts, and even meat and dairy—serves as a powerful energy source. Your body burns good fat as fuel, which helps power up your brain as well as the rest of your system. Fat also slows the rate at which your body digests the rest of your food, helping you feel satiated and avoid the kind of blood sugar fluctuations that rev your appetite and make you feel shaky and off-kilter.

Even more important, fat makes up your cell membranes, and you have a lot of cells. Every cell—no matter what kind— is made of lipids, which is to say fat, and has two layers of fatty acids. Your body uses the fat you consume to make these cell membranes. If you consume too little fat, your tissues and organs don't function properly because your cell membranes aren't being "fed." In fact, a wealth of new research shows that a high-fat, low-carbohydrate diet improves the function of mitochondria— that is, the tiny energy-revving system within each of your cells. Healthy mitochondria improve overall health at the cellular level and increase life span—which helps explain why new research from the UC Davis School of Veterinary Medicine found that mice fed a high-fat diet outlived those that consumed less fat.[5]

Fat Fruit

Chinese medicine has used mulberry tree fruit and bark for literally thousands of years to treat circulatory diseases like heart disease, diabetes, anemia, and arthritis. The linoleic acids, available in the mulberry fruit and the slippery inner bark, both optimize hydration and help absorb fat-soluble nutrients from our diets. Mulberry tea is served throughout Asia in the late afternoons, when hydration levels so often decline.[6] Mulberries are also native to the eastern United States and were used in Native American medicines, also, as in the Chinese traditions, both bark and berry.

Fat doesn't deserve its bad rap. One series of studies published in the *Journal of the American Medical Association* showed that women who got 32 percent of their calories from fat had the same rates of breast and colon cancers, heart attacks, and strokes as those whose diets contained 20 percent fat.[7] In fact, several new studies, including the Prospective Urban Rural Epidemiology project, are finding that a higher intake of unsaturated and saturated fat (that's no typo) is tied to better health. A high-carbohydrate diet, on the other hand, ups your odds of conditions like heart disease, diabetes, and obesity.[8] In Dana's work as a physician, she's seen thousands of people lose weight, improve their blood pressure and cholesterol, and turn their health around by following a low-carb diet that's plentiful in healthy fats.[9]

Fat serves another important purpose: It helps your body absorb health-boosting, disease-fighting, fat-soluble vitamins, including A, D, E, and K. To wit: One study from Ohio State University showed that people who ate salsa prepared with avocado absorbed four times more lycopene from tomatoes and nearly three times more vitamin A than those who had a version made without avocado.[10]

If that isn't reason enough to start saying yes to fat, Dr. Gerald Pollack's lab tests have shown that ghee—that is, clarified butter, which happens to be a healthful form of fat—is loaded with ultrahydrating water, hinting at the possibility that other forms of fat may play a crucial role in hydration. It may also explain why camels' humps are made of fat—yes, fat!—rather than water, as most of us have been led to believe. It makes you wonder if fat plays a role in their legendary ability to travel in hot conditions for mile after mile without a water source.

If you're eating egg whites for breakfast, a salad topped with lean turkey and fat-free dressing for lunch, and pasta with tomato sauce for dinner, you'll probably be happy to know that adding some extra flavor—in the form of egg yolks, a drizzle of olive oil, and even some red meat and cheese—may also improve your health and up your ability to hydrate optimally.

But doesn't eating fat make you fat?

You've heard it a million times: Dietary fat converts to body fat faster than carbohydrates and protein. It's a myth. While fat does pack more than double the calories found in protein and carbohydrates (nine calories in fat versus four calories in protein and carbs), including a moderate amount in your diet won't stall your weight-loss efforts. In fact, research shows that increasing your intake may actually help you slim down. A recent study from Stanford University found that people who got around 40 percent of their calories from fat lost twice as much weight as those who got about 20 percent of total calories from fat over the course of eight weeks.[11]

Why? Fat makes your stomach digest food more slowly, so you to feel fuller, longer. It's safe to say that you can slim down just by upping your water intake and adding a serving of healthy fat, like half an avocado or some olive oil, each meal. That's why very low-fat diets can be so hard to follow—even if you're taking in enough calories, you may experience nagging feelings of hunger, prompting you to overeat later or blow off your diet altogether.

NOT ALL FATS ARE CREATED EQUAL

Most fats are actually a mixture of fatty acids. The majority of the time, they're defined by the fatty acid they have the most of, such as saturated, polyunsaturated, and so on. As you probably know, there are two primary groups of fats: unsaturated and saturated. Here's how they differ.

Unsaturated fats are a type of fat having a high proportion of fatty acid molecules with at least one double bond. All unsaturated fat is good for you. But the two types, monounsaturated and polyunsaturated, are healthy for different reasons.

Monounsaturated fat is found in seeds, plants, and plant oils like olive oil as well as avocados, pumpkin seeds, and peanuts.

All monounsaturated fats are omega-9 fatty acids. They get their name from the first double bond on the fatty acid chain, and they've been shown to decrease the risk of cardiovascular disease. The superstar of this fat category is olive oil, which has a high concentration of monounsaturated fat and is teeming with oleic acid—a type of omega-9 that has particularly heart-protective effects.

Don't run to the grocery store and grab any old olive oil, though. Choose extra-virgin, which means it was pressed without chemicals. We also recommend cold-pressed, organic oil, which ensures the oil was protected from light, thereby reducing oxidation during the pressing process. Pressing within six hours of harvesting leads to the highest concentration of nutrients. Consider macadamia nut oil, too. It's even higher in monounsaturated fat than olive oil, and though it can be pricy, its very high smoke point (413 degrees Fahrenheit) and delicious buttery flavor make it the unsung hero of the cooking oil realm.

Polyunsaturated fats are found in plant oils like safflower, corn, soybean, and sunflower oil, certain nuts like walnuts, and fatty fish like salmon and sardines, as well as grass-fed red meat and free-range eggs.

There are two types of polyunsaturated fats: omega-3 and omega-6 fatty acids. A wealth of research shows that omega-3 fatty acids are especially important for our health—and you have to get them from food, because your body can't make them on its own. Omega-3-rich foods include fatty fish like salmon, tuna, and sardines, flaxseed, chia, walnuts, free-range eggs, and grass-fed red meat.

Over the past two decades, research shows that omega-3s play a role in everything from lowering blood pressure and balancing cholesterol to fighting age-related memory loss and Alzheimer's disease. Some experts even say that omega-3 fatty acids can improve your mood and defend against depression. They're nutritional powerhouses—not only does your body absorb them more easily than other kinds of fat, but once they're in your cells, they reduce inflammation that leads to chronic health conditions. For example, a review of forty-six separate studies from researchers at Tufts University found that people who increased their intake of the omega-3 fatty acids EPA and DHA from supplements and/or fish had a reduced risk of cardiac arrest and death from all causes.

There are different types of omega-3s, and they have different effects. While all three main varieties—ALA, DHA, and EPA—have a positive impact on your health, the latter two are more potent disease fighters. ALA comes from plant sources, like vegetables and seeds, including chia; while DHA and EPA come from marine sources, including seafood and algae. If you're not a fan of fillets, opt for fish oil capsules, or go for a DHA supplement made from algae or krill oil, which are less taxing on our ocean environment.

As for omega-6s, they're healthy, too—especially a type of omega-6 called GLA, which is found in evening primrose and borage oil. These are the ones important for making our sex hormones. In her practice, Dana often sees young women with amenorrhea—their period stops. She finds that replacing these fats by adding either a supplement or increasing the fat in their diets does the trick. Their periods miraculously return with no other interventions. This is a more common problem than you would expect, and we are not talking about the eating-disorder patients who lose their periods. Many people still subscribe to the low-fat-diet lifestyle.

Omega-6s also happen to be the most common type of fatty acids in the American diet. And because of that, most of us get too many omega-6s and too few omega-3s, which keeps us from deriving the maximum health benefits you get from having the right balance of omega-3s, -6s, and -9s. It's one more reason to limit your intake of processed food—much of which is loaded with omega-6s—and make a point to get omega-3s from whole-food sources like salmon, walnuts, and ground chia seed.

SATURATED FAT

Saturated fat is a type of fat that's mostly found in animal foods and, in lesser degrees, certain other foods like coconut. It's different from unsaturated fat, because each of its carbon atoms are loaded with a hydrogen molecule, which forms a straight chain. Unsaturated fat, on the other hand, has at least one "bend" in the chain. Most of the time, it becomes solid at room temperature and liquefies in heat—think coconut oil and butter.

For years, health experts claimed that saturated fat was a serious risk factor in heart disease and obesity, among other health conditions. But in the past decade, the tide has begun to turn. Among other evidence, a randomized control study—that's the gold standard of studies—of forty-six overweight men in the *American Journal of Clinical Nutrition* found that those who followed a high-fat diet actually *improved* their health: The high-fat regime resulted in lower blood pressure, a reduction in belly fat, and better insulin and blood sugar control.

Skipping saturated fat altogether is bad for your brain. Your brain's white matter contains phospholipids—those are a type of fat that are a major component of all cell membranes. Phospholipids play a role in numerous metabolic processes, and they're made of both saturated and monounsaturated fat. Because your body can't make saturated fat, you have to eat it in order to "feed" your phospholipids and keep your brain healthy.

It's not just research, though—go on any website or blog about Paleo-style diets and you'll find legions of people who found that more protein and saturated fat and fewer carbohydrates gave them more energy, better health, and a leaner waistline.

Controversy remains: The National Institutes of Health still recommend swapping saturated fat for monounsaturated vegetable oils, and some questions about saturated fat still need to be answered. We think the problem lies in the fact that the majority of research on saturated fat doesn't separate the different types (more on that shortly).

But it's safe to say that if you're focused on cutting out saturated fat but still carb-loading pasta, bread, and sugar, you're missing the forest for the trees. A healthy body requires a whole-health diet that centers on unprocessed food—and yes, plenty of water.

THE BEST KIND OF SATURATED FAT

At the risk of sounding like a broken record, saturated fats—like all other fats—aren't all the same. Instead, they can be broken up into categories based on how long their molecules are.

Some of the healthiest saturated fats are **short-chain fatty acids (SCFAs)**. They're the type found in butter, ghee, and high-fat dairy. These forms of saturated fat are particularly high in butyrate, an SCFA that protects against colon cancer, serves as a potent form of energy for the cells in your gastrointestinal tract, and even reduces inflammation, making it important for preventing and treating autoimmune diseases. Early research shows that SCFAs may improve metabolism, spurring weight loss.

DR. DANA'S CASE STUDY

Lisa

Lisa, a forty-nine-year-old copywriter at an advertising firm, had come to me with a host of issues from Sjögren's disease, an autoimmune disorder that, among other symptoms, causes arthritis and dry eyes and mouth as it dehydrates the body's moisture-producing glands. She was distressed by her chronically and sometimes painfully dry eyes and skin, which sometimes tightened around her joints. And she had fatigue that was interfering with her work and keeping her from the gym and socializing. With tears in her eyes, she told me about how rheumatologist after rheumatologist had told her that her condition would only get worse as she aged and that drugs or steroids were the only course of treatment—that and saline solution. But long-term steroid use has serious drawbacks, such as diabetes and osteoporosis, and Lisa was rightfully concerned.

I wanted to provide her some relief, and with dehydration playing a big part in her condition, I asked if she'd like to try to hydrate better as a first step. She first nodded but then looked hesitant. "Will this be a lot of work?" she asked. She was already overworked, and a complicated plan would overwhelm her. I could feel her stress palpably as she talked. "Overwork can dehydrate," I said, and I could see tears forming. I reassured her that it would be easy to integrate into her busy routine.

She first asked if she'd have to give up coffee. She lived on caffeine for fuel—at least five cups of coffee a day. Caffeine at that level is a mild diuretic, so it dehydrates No, I told her, she wouldn't have to go cold turkey, but she would have to lessen the load. And the easiest way to do that was with ghee. "*Ghee?*" she asked. Yup, ghee. Ghee is a type of fat that increases long-lasting energy while slowing the absorption of caffeine. That meant she wouldn't need five cups to get through her morning, let alone her whole day. Ghee also improves cognition and reduces brain fog.

We laid out a three-week program, including the jump start plan, then two more weeks of hydrating meals consisting of two vegetables with each meal. Lisa's typical workday consisted of sitting in front of a computer for many hours at a time, often eating lunch at her desk. So she needed a better balanced lunch menu—no more Amy's frozen burritos, her fallback meal, which had about 20 percent of her total daily recommended sodium content. Frozen foods are often overloaded with salt. She had hoped she could replace her drink of choice—Coke—with juice.

"Isn't juice hydrating?" she asked.

I told her that unfortunately juice has as much sugar as soda, but she could drink smoothies that are core to the Quench Plan. She lit up—there was a smoothie place right near her office. Together we reviewed the menu online and wrote out a five-day lunch plan.

For exercise, I gave her some simple micromovements to do while she commuted on the subway, like neck swirls and ankle swirls. I also gave her some breathing techniques to do when she was stressed, along with simple stretches and walkabouts she could do at her desk. She had been somewhat familiar with desk yoga, but it was a revelation to her that the movements would help move fluid through her body.

We agreed to have a check-in after three weeks. When Lisa returned, I could clearly see change: She beamed and spoke with more energy. She talked about feeling less depressed and not as overwhelmed. And the symptoms of her Sjögren's disease had lessened, as well—she was down to using less than half the amount of the saline eye drops she had before (she had previously gone through a small bottle a day), and her skin and lips were no longer scaly. She said she didn't get that afternoon fatigue any-more. She was going out twice a week. She had even lost three pounds!

With such great results in hand, we designed a longer-term plan that included a variety of smoothies so she wouldn't get bored while getting her optimum hydration. Some of those other variet-ies are found in the recipe section of this book. In addition, I gave her a bone broth recipe and recommended she drink broth instead of that midmorning coffee she was used to. Lisa continues to stay hydrated, and her symptoms remain at bay.

Another healthful type of saturated fat is **medium chain fatty acids**, which are also known as **medium chain triglyc-erides (MCTs)**. Butter contains some MCTs, but coconut oil and palm kernel oil have higher concentrations. There's a rea-son why many health-conscious folks sing the praises of coco-nut oil: Research shows that MCTs boost metabolism, improve insulin sensitivity, and even help improve critical thinking and memory.

Last, there are **long chain fatty acids (LCFAs)** and **very long chain fatty acids (VLCFAs)**, both of which are found in most animal foods (though these acids are also found in mono-unsaturated and polyunsaturated fat, too). While not the health foe that they've long been claimed to be, they have fewer health benefits than SCFAs and MCTs. One main reason is their inability to cross the blood-brain barrier—which is to say, your brain can't use them as fuel.

LCFAs are abundant in the American diet, particularly in processed oils that have gone rancid from light exposure or from being overheated, and in lard from meat and dairy products made from non-grass-fed animals. That's why we recommend choosing lean cuts, trimming the fat off red meat, and choosing fish and poultry more often.

WHAT ABOUT COOKING OIL?

When it comes to choosing an oil to cook with, there are myriad options: canola, olive, coconut, peanut, avocado, soybean—and many more.

The first thing to think about when considering an oil is its smoke point. That's the temperature at which the oil starts to smoke. Put simply, the higher the smoke point, the better. When an oil begins to smoke, it starts to oxidize and release unhealthy trans fats. That's also the point at which it becomes unstable and releases health-harming molecules like aldehydes and alcohols. This process is called lipid peroxidation—and in addition to making food taste bad, it causes cellular damage that contributes to a host of diseases like asthma, Parkinson's, and inflammatory bowel disease, to name a few.[12]

Healthy cooking oil options with high smoke points happen to be chock-full of plant-healthy compounds, including:

- Avocado oil
- Peanut oil—Notably, it has a neutral flavor and doesn't contain allergy-causing peanut protein. Please ask your allergist first if you have a severe peanut allergy!
- Coconut oil—It tends to have a strong coconut flavor.
- Extra-virgin olive oil—The healthiest choice, it has a slightly lower smoke point, so use it while cooking at temperatures less than 320 degrees Fahrenheit—or best just drizzle it on your food once it's done cooking.
- Macadamia nut oil—It's delicious and neutral in flavor, but pricy.
- Ghee
- Grapeseed oil
- Sesame oil

Important: While flaxseed is healthful, save it for dressing salads and adding to smoothies, and *never* cook with it or heat it—doing so can quickly cause the release of damaging lipid peroxides.

You may be wondering, *What about canola oil?* It's ubiquitous in cooking sprays and recipes that call for oil. While it has a high smoke point and is made of monounsaturated fat, most canola oils and canola products are genetically modified. And the vast majority of canola oil, which comes from the rapeseed, a flowering, bright yellow member of the mustard and cabbage family, is sprayed with pesticides right before harvest. Given what we know about the connection between pesticides and health problems like cancer and metabolic syndrome, canola oil suddenly looks like a less than healthy choice.

A Quick and Dirty Guide to Choosing the Right Fat

Eat a varied diet full of fresh, whole food and you won't have to obsess about whether you're eating too much fat or choosing the right kinds. It's really that easy: By opting for "real" food rather than the kind that comes in a box or microwavable package, you'll avoid unhealthy trans fat. We know the hydrogenated kind that's been tied to countless health problems, from obesity to diabetes to stroke. Stay away from less healthy fats like lard that are abundant in processed foods like chips, cookies, muffins, and snack crackers.

Fats have more to do with hydration that we ever suspected, so let's say good-bye to the days of fat phobia and make the right decisions about adding fats back into our diet. In this case, oil and water *do* mix.

CHAPTER 6

Who Needs Water the Most?

Ideal Hydration for High-Need Populations

The cure for anything is salt water: sweat, tears or the sea.

—*Isak Dinesen*

While everyone needs to be much more aware of the importance of hydration, there are those who have to pay particular attention: children, athletes, and the elderly. For our kids, hydration is critical to their growing bodies and minds. For athletes, hydrating properly will help them perform better, stronger, faster—and better avoid concussion and injury. And for the elderly, hydration is harder to maintain, because as we age, the water content in our body decreases, and thus the potential for dehydration increases. Let's take a deeper dive into how we can ensure that our loved ones get the water they need.

CHILDREN

Children are particularly susceptible to dehydration, because their growing bodies need water to develop and mature. Infants, especially, can become dehydrated only hours after becoming ill, and dehydration is a major cause of infant illness and death throughout the world.

And for older kids, all that running around and play means they lose large amounts of water. Children also tend not to drink enough water to make up the loss. Any mother would tell you their children have to be reminded to drink—they are just too busy playing! If a recent Harvard T. H. Chan School of Public Health study is to be believed, more than half of all children and adolescents in the United States are not getting enough hydration. Hydration has important consequences for their still-forming physical, cognitive, and emotional functions. Interestingly, the study also found that black children have a higher risk of dehydration than white children. Also, boys have a higher risk than girls. And surprisingly, nearly 25 percent of children report that they drink no plain water at all. It makes you wonder what the heck they are drinking, if anything.

Although it can be hard to get kids to drink in school, there are some great ways to ensure kids are getting proper hydration. Take, for instance, the Hydration Pilot Project at the Ideal School, run in collaboration with the Hydration Foundation. It took place over a year in 2014 in an independent school in Manhattan. The staff drew up an "oasis" map of the school to find out where water fountains and other sources of water were placed. Based on the map, the school staff were better able to see where there wasn't easy and ample access to water, and as a solution they brought in water pitchers to classrooms. Were there spills? You bet. Were there better test scores? Yes. They also made sure kids hydrated before and after gym class. And in a surprise finding, the more access to drinking water kids had, the easier behavior management became. Afternoon focus became discernably improved. And after school coaches sent kids into games pre-protected by hydration from injury. With every student taking a planned water break, it became a part of the school culture, and it also set the stage for kids to grow up to drink water regularly.

Phones Dehydrate

We are all on our phones, either looking at screens or carrying on conversations. We look at our phones to keep updated on Facebook and Twitter, get directions, and tell someone we are going to be late. Adolescents are especially glued to their phones. But did you know that scrolling through your cell phone is dehydrating? There are two reasons for this: First, we have to manufacture a new round of neurochemicals, using up hydration, every time we refocus. All that looking up and down and interruption costs us as we draw on our nutrition and water reserves to resynthesize and reproduce the next round of focus chemicals. Second, if your head is down and tipped forward, that added pressure on your neck means the synovial fluid, passing to your brain from your spinal canal, is compressed and slowed in its flow. Each use may diminish and deplete only a small percentage, but it's happening repeatedly through the day. See the Quench Plan for our simple micromovements that restores flow for cell phone users!

When a friend of Gina's was struggling with her child's attention deficit hyperactivity disorder, particularly getting him to focus in school, Gina told her about the Hydration Pilot Project. Based on the success of this pilot, the mother went to her own son's teacher and shared the results. Sure enough, the teacher implemented some of these new strategies. Specifically, instead of asking the child to try to focus over and over again, she would send him out for a drink at the fountain. He would come back from that short break better able to work.

His focus and behavior have since remarkably improved. Why? Because the child was getting more hydration and moving more. This is a beautiful example of how hydration and movement can increase focus when paired.

In the pilot study, when staff from the Hydration Foundation explained to the students that water conducted electricity and was therefore necessary for getting more electricity to the brain, students were fascinated and drank more willingly and with intention to focus on schoolwork. During one art class a student asked for a drink so her artwork "would come out better." They clearly made the connection between drinking and getting themselves focused to work.[1] Smart kids!

The good news is that the public health problem of children and dehydration has a simple solution, concludes Steven Gortmaker, professor of health sociology at Harvard. "If we can focus on helping children drink more water—a low-cost, no-calorie beverage—we can improve their hydration status, which may allow many children to feel better throughout the day and do better in school."[2]

We see an even better solution. Where typical school snacks such as crackers, pretzels, or granola bars add to the problem, replace these with fresh water-rich foods such as apple slices, cucumber slices, celery, peaches, cantaloupe, strawberries, and grapes—as well as the smoothies and fruit popsicles from the Quench Plan! In preschools, young ones love helping make fruit platters. Let them be creative with what fruits to use, and have them come up with names for the concoctions.

THE ATHLETE AND WEEKEND WARRIORS

Sports and exercise should be a part of your daily routine. Some work out a little more than others, and some sweat a little more than others. Some sweat a *lot* more. And gym junkies need to be extra careful about hydration. And we are talking about you, Bikram yoga people. Boy, do you sweat. Here's why that's wonderful.

Sweat gets no respect. Yet it is a crucial, delicately complicated outflow system, collaborating with many other body networks. It takes energy to sweat, and it's a complex process. Depending on your body's resting metabolic rate (that is, how many calories you burn at rest), your kidneys alone can burn more than four hundred calories a day—and much of that energy is spent balancing your body's fluid intake between cells and organs.[3]

Sweating is an essential component of your body's internal thermostat; it allows you to cool down fast, which keeps your organs, blood, and tissues from overheating.[4] Sweating is one of the many ways your body naturally detoxifies; it helps remove certain compounds from your bloodstream. It's also the delivery system for your natural pheromones—scented "sex hormones" that influence whom you attract and whom you're attracted to.[5]

Sweat is produced in glands that are located in your skin's dermis—the layer directly underneath the part of your skin you can touch. While you have sweat glands all over your body, the forehead, armpits, palms, and soles of your feet are likely to have the highest concentration.

SO . . . WHAT IS IT, EXACTLY?

The exact composition of sweat varies from person to person and from day to day. But it's approximately 99 percent water. What's in the other 1 percent? The electrolytes sodium and chloride, as well as ammonia, sugar, and very small amounts of minerals like calcium, potassium, magnesium, iron, zinc, copper, and certain water-soluble vitamins.[6] In order to properly replenish what we lose through sweat, we need not only to replace water but to replace electrolytes. Adding some natural sea salt to our water bottles addresses this beautifully.

REPLENISHING AFTER A SWEAT SESSION

Certain things you can't entirely control—like menopause, stress, and preperformance jitters—can trigger sweating. Genetics and health conditions can play a role in how much you sweat. Ditto for weight: The more you weigh, the harder your body has to work to stay cool, which leads to extra sweat.

Still, the amount you sweat is most directly tied to your physical activity levels. If you're doing light exercise like walking or biking comfortably, in a cool or moderate-temperature space, you might sweat as little as one hundred milliliters, or three ounces, in an hour. If you're doing vigorous exercise such as running at a fast pace, and in a warm or hot environment, you might lose more than three thousand milliliters, or one hundred ounces, of sweat in over an hour.[7]

As a general guideline, Tim Coyle, an exercise physiologist in Dana's office, recommends the following to adequately replenish:

- Drink four to eight ounces of water for every fifteen minutes of activity during the activity. Use thirst as your guide, but be careful not to chug more than twelve ounces of water every fifteen minutes; you run the risk of overhydrating.
- If you're doing an extreme sport, like running a marathon or training, drink about 2.5 cups (or 20 ounces) of water 2.5 hours before exercise, and then another 1.5 cups (or 12 ounces) 15 minutes before exercise. This ensures you don't dehydrate while you're exercising.

It may take some trial and error to figure out what's right for you. Another fairly simple way to tell if you're healthfully hydrating for your workouts: Step on a scale before you begin, and then again when you're done. According to the American College of Sports Medicine, an increase or decrease in weight can indicate if you have enough fluid in your system.

- **Well-hydrated:** −1 to + 1 percent change in your body weight—for example, if you're 150 pounds, you would neither lose nor gain more than 1.5 pounds immediately following a workout.
- **Slightly dehydrated:** −1 to −3 percent—if you're 150 pounds, you'd lose 1.5 to 4.5 pounds immediately following a workout.
- **Significantly dehydrated:** −3 to −5 percent—if you're 150 pounds, you'd lose 4.5 to 7.5 pounds immediately following a workout.
- **Seriously dehydrated:** −5 percent or more—if you're 150 pounds, you'd lose 7.5 pounds or more immediately following a workout.[8]

LET THIRST BE YOUR GUIDE—TO A POINT

While the adage "Let thirst be your guide" is generally good advice, you have to be careful not to let thirst trick you into drinking too much water—especially during and after a heavy bout of exercise, like a triathlon, or when you're in extreme heat. Overhydrating can lead to a condition called hyponatremia, which occurs when the sodium levels in your blood become critically low because you have too much water running through your system. This causes your cells to swell, and it can cause serious problems and can even be life-threatening.[9] An estimated 13 percent of people who compete in the Boston Marathon develop hyponatremia, which is one of the many reasons medical professionals are on hand to assist runners.[10]

Dehydration and Heat Disorders

The first signs of dehydration may include increased thirst, dizziness, weakness, fatigue, headache, dry skin, dry mouth, fatigue, and amber-colored or concentrated urine or less urine output. More severe dehydration can present with anuria (no urine output), dizziness that renders the person unable to stand or walk normally, low blood pressure, fast heart rate, fever, lethargy, and confusion, and it can lead to seizures, shock, or coma. These symptoms require immediate medical attention.

For those who are dehydrated and vomiting, try to get them to sip water slowly or suck on popsicles made from juice or electrolyte drinks. In those who are dehydrated and not vomiting, an effective and immediate treatment for dehydration is to replace lost fluids with cool water containing a pinch of salt. Also cool the body with a wet towel or mist the person's skin with water from a spray bottle. If it is an emergency, grab a sports drink or a Pedialyte. This level of dehydration is no time to worry about details like sugar consumption. Hydration is urgent and critical.

Three heat syndromes related to dehydration are heat cramps, heat exhaustion, and heat stroke. **Heat cramps** are painful, brief muscle cramps also known as charley horses. They are caused by losing electrolytes through heavy exertion and not properly replacing them. They can occur in the calves, thighs, abdomen, and shoulders. **Heat exhaustion** is preventable, and the symptoms include cool skin, heavy sweating, feeling faint, light-headedness, fatigue, weakness, fast heart rate, low blood pressure upon standing, muscle cramps, nausea, and headache. It can be prevented by hydrating properly during exercise, wearing proper lightweight clothing, and watching the temperatures outside and not exercising when the heat index is high. Heat exhaustion, if left untreated, can lead to **heat stroke**, which is a life-threatening condition that requires immediate medical attention. Its telltale sign is a fever of more than 104 degrees.

WHAT ABOUT SPORTS DRINKS?

While advertisers would love for you to think otherwise, you don't need to down a Gatorade after spending half an hour on the elliptical or twenty minutes lifting weights. Provided you're not skimping on sodium and are choosing a diet filled with fresh food, your body can balance its electrolytes after "normal" exercise. A glass of water—not a special sports drink—will work just fine to quench your thirst and replenish your water stores.

If you're exercising over an hour, it's a good idea to eat and/or drink something that provides glucose (i.e., fuel) in the form of carbohydrates and electrolytes (particularly sodium). Dana advises endurance athlete clients to steer clear of any beverage loaded with artificial colors and added sugar and instead choose our following DIY drink.

SIP SMARTER: DIY SPORTS DRINK

You can replenish your electrolytes, water, and carbohydrates with this beverage, which only contains natural ingredients.

- 8 to 12 ounces of plain or coconut water
- A pinch of natural salt (like sea or Celtic)
- A squirt (about 0.5 to 1 ounce) of lemon or lime juice
- A teaspoon of honey or maple syrup

AFTER-SCHOOL SPORTS

Here is why hydrating—and with a little salt, essential electrolytes, too—is crucial after school for young athletes: injury protection. Rethink hydration as simply replacing fluids, and imagine how it buffers tissues and cells. Water, ever blessing, is not only providing energy but providing sponginess, right as young athletes are going into all sorts of contact. Hydrating late in the day is not only essential for staying brain smart through those last hours of a school day (and by the way, can anyone explain why chemistry is always the last class of the day for high schoolers?), but for those kids with after-school sports, hydrating is concussion and tissue protective.

We don't want to scare you with statistics on young-athlete

concussions and the hidden but lasting consequences, so we will cut straight to the solution. Hydration is the first and foremost way to preprotect and preload, offering muscle and brain buffering. And if you couple it with oils, especially omega-3s, you have strategically sent in the inner-body defense team, all ready to repel injury or concussion. The evidence on preprotecting the brain and treating concussions with omega-3s is now legion. The research was initiated by the U.S. Army. Dr. Michael Lewis, a former colonel with the U.S. Army Medical Corps, documented how omega-3 supplementation prior to brain injury could protect, and speed recovery, if injury occurred.[11]

How about a sports drink that accomplishes that? A drink that delivers hydration, electrolytes and omega-3s in one guzzle? We developed a Quench recipe just for that and named it the Tara Fix (see the following recipe) to honor the ancient tribe of the Tarahumara, made famous in the book we mentioned earlier, *Born to Run*. They fuel all that running with chia seeds, so we are right back to where we started the Quench research: Alternative hydrating strategies abound in many cultures. Desert peoples have so much to share about hydration.

Tara Fix

ONE SERVING

12 oz water

1 or 2 teaspoons ground chia seeds (omega-3s)

4 oz kombucha, your favorite flavor; ginger is great. The Tarahumara mixed chia with their homemade fermented corn beer. Kombucha is our substitute.

1 pinch sea or rock salt

Combine the ingredients in a water bottle. Cap the bottle, shake vigorously, and enjoy.

Desert Peoples' Lack of Fish

Omega-3 oils are most potently found in fish. But what if your tribe has no access to fish? Evolutionary adaption to environments enables desert dwellers to convert ALA, found in seeds, nuts, or even algae from seasonal lakes, more efficiently into EPA and DHA. Remember, most desert peoples are nomadic. Tribes in central Africa would gather in the spring all around Lake Victoria. Anthropologists recorded mostly all the marriage contracts, feasting, dancing, and celebrating they did during these large seasonal gatherings. But guess what? Along with all that partying, the women were gathering algae from the lake, drying it, and packing it up to make it through the next hardship season. There you have it: omega-3s in the diet from algae.

For us, getting your omega-3s from fish or even store-bought krill oil is more likely. But we can't say enough about how important omega-3 intake is. Just know that other peoples in other times would travel great distances at great effort to get some in their diet. And for the vegan among us, explore coupling your ALA intake (typically through flaxseeds, walnuts, or chia) with coconut oil, which may help in convert ALA into EPA and DHA more efficiently.

WORKPLACE ATHLETES

For most of us, work is an athletic event. Keeping cool, alert, flexible, with snap-ready responses, is just as athletic as being out on the field. Work environments are notorious for drying us up. Let's rethink our day as an athletic one, using all our new tricks, slipping in micromovements as an everyday habit. Even big-building corporations are slowly catching on. A large bank recently took away personal trash cans from their employees, not as a punitive measure but to get them to get up and move! But you don't need your employer to make your workday athletic. Choose yourself to be a workday warrior instead of just a weekend one. Micromove and hydrate like you would at the gym.

HYDRATION AND THE ELDERLY

With age, hydration has consequences far more pronounced. According to Barry Popkin, an expert in dehydration, our thirst mechanism diminishes with age, which coincides with our loss of muscle.[12] Muscle tissue is one of the largest places we bank our water, so our ability to *store* water declines right around the same time as our body's signal to drink. This is a double whammy, resulting in frequent urinary tract infections, gastrointestinal distress, loss of cognitive powers, confusion, fatigue, balance loss, and a cascade of consequences—all of which can be intercepted by adequate hydration. And snowbirds—seniors who relocate to warmer climates for the winter or permanently—are also more susceptible in warmer weather to becoming dehydrated.

DR. DANA'S CASE STUDY

Havie

One of my patients, Havie, is a seventy-four-year-old fashion designer who is amazingly energetic and active for her age. The only thing that slows her down is the osteoarthritis in her neck. She had neck surgery more than fifteen years ago, but her whole upper carriage bothers her. She has seen orthopedists, chiropractors, physical therapists, acupuncturists, and massage therapists. She takes ibuprofen fairly regularly and needs to push herself through the pain to get through her day.

Also, after having an endoscopy a year ago that showed she had a hiatal hernia, she had been prescribed omeprazole—a proton pump inhibitor. She religiously takes the medication every day, and while it has helped, she has a bitterness in her mouth as well as unpleasant, thick phlegm. She also felt pressure in her chest, but she had seen a cardiologist, and all of her tests had come back normal.

Besides taking over-the-counter pain medication and the inhaler, she takes a cholesterol-lowering drug (Zetia), even though she had no history of heart disease: Her doctor had put her on it years ago as a preventative measure, because her cholesterol levels were "borderline high."

After getting her medical history, I asked her about her typical diet, which consisted of the following.

Breakfast: Coffee, sometimes two cups. She never eats breakfast during the week; on weekends she may have granola and yogurt or eggs.

Lunch: Salad, sometimes with grilled chicken, and Snapple iced tea.

Dinner: Salmon and veggies, water. It's rare for her to have dessert.

I asked her if she thought she drank enough water.

"Probably not," she replied. "If I drink too much, I have to pee all day!"

"I'd like for you to hydrate yourself better as a first step," I said. "Let's get you off needless medications and give you a better diet."

When I described some of the possible side effects of even the most benign drug like omeprazole—which includes joint pain and reflux—and explained that they might even be contributing to her pain and fatigue, she agreed she wanted off of them.

I started Havie on a Quench jump start program while we waited for the initial blood work to come back. While her diet was good, I had her make some easy tweaks. She needed to drink a glass of water before every meal, but her mornings needed the most work. Instead of skipping breakfast, she needed to start her day with a smoothie, along with a large glass of water with lemon and a pinch of sea salt.

With that suggestion Havie was shocked. "I had always thought salt was bad for me, and I avoided it like the plague!"

I explained, "There's difference between good salt like sea salt, loaded with minerals, and the girl-with-the-umbrella salt, which is best used on your icy driveway."

I also added the afternoon smoothie for additional hydration, as I suspected her meal portions were very small and she would do well with the added smoothie.

Because of her neck pain, we added some micromovements as a course of action. I had her do some morning stretching while lying in bed, like the Chin Meets Chest (see chapter 8) and the Full Body Stretch, described in the Quench Plan. I also gave her some simple stretches throughout the day, like gently nodding her head every time she got into an elevator and doing simple shoulder lifts.

Havie came back to my office for a check-in three weeks later. She looked gorgeous. There was a sparkle in her eyes.

"How are you feeling?" I asked.

"I haven't felt this good in ten years. My stiffness is so much better," she replied.

"How much better?"

"Eighty percent better! I still need to take Tylenol every morning, but I haven't needed to take any omeprazole in two weeks. My reflux is completely gone. The bitter taste in my mouth—gone. The thick mucus—gone!"

Her lab work had come back, and everything was normal, except her vitamin D was a little low and her total cholesterol was 160—way *below* normal levels. I was so happy to be able to take Havie off her cholesterol-lowering drug and see how the Quench Plan worked for her in the long run. She wholeheartedly agreed.

By Havie's six-month checkup, the Quench Plan had become routine. Now that she was off the medications, her cholesterol came back at 190—still below normal. Every morning she makes smoothies for herself and her husband. Her shoulders and neck are remarkably better, with a much greater range on motion. She continues to use Tylenol for pain, but not every day. She also told me that she now takes the stairs to her third-floor apartment and continues to do her neck exercises in the morning and in the elevator. By hydrating wiser with food and movement, she became more fluid with less pain and less drugs, and that bad taste in her mouth mysteriously disappeared.

As I suspected, when she became better and wiser about hydration—using hydrating foods and water along with movement—the joints and muscles in her shoulders, arms, and neck became better lubricated, and her pain markedly decreased. As a result, she is continuing these nutrition and lifestyle changes for the long term.

Medication is a risk factor as well, as older people tend to take more medication for a variety of conditions. This simultaneous use of drugs, believe it or not, has a name: polypharmacy. Lee Hooper, Diane Bunn, and Suzan Whitelock, all research nurses, were the first to conduct a study that measured how polypharmacy affected dehydration among the elderly.[13] They noted that caretakers need to be vigilant as to whether their patients are drinking enough and take steps to help them drink more. There are logistics that complicate the issue, such as the patients' mobility and their concern about reaching the bathroom in time. Our elders may also suffer from their physical inability to make or to reach drinks or have swallowing issues, which is common. One ridiculously simple trick to double hydration for the elderly, or anyone, is to use two straws to sip a drink instead of one. Gina used to tape two straws together to make it easier for her mom to get more with each sip. Larger straws often used for bubble tea can also help.

The Rose

Traditions exist the world over for the rose's healing powers. Roses were originally raised for their medicinal applications, and their beauty is an added benefit. Ancient recipes from Persia to India typically created sweetened jams and jellies from the high pectin content in the petals. Roses' hydrating effects were put into practice to address overexposure to heat, fatigue, and all the symptoms typically associated with dehydration, such as head and muscle aches, dry eye, dizziness, and cognitive fog. Called Gulkand across the Indian subcontinent, it is a common staple in traditional pantries. Typically *Rosa damascena*, more commonly known as the

Damascus rose, was further used for its purifying properties and for helping memory. By the very early Middle Ages, the Apothecary rose, *Rosa gallica*, was found in every herbal manuscript and recorded among the inventory of plants common to medicinal gardens. Rose teas became common and a pleasure, but for the real hydrating power, use of its absorptive pectin was advised.

And did you know that ancient Persians from Kashan used rose jelly to heal their ill? The jelly was made from the high pectin content of the rose petals, which aided tissue moisture. Ancient Persian doctors used rose petal jam especially for the elderly, slipping it under their tongues to release both the high-pectin hydration and the medicinal effects locked within, in the gentlest possible release. Rose jelly was especially noted to heal mucous membranes, which line our digestive tract. Mucus requires hydration to form. In fact, rose petals in Persia were grown in herb gardens along with other plants to be used for pharmacological interventions. Immortalized for their beauty, we've forgotten their medicinal agents, yet now modern science[14] has tested the medicinal elements of rose petals, and experiments have shown bacteria died within five minutes of contact with fresh rose petals. Roses have been shown to have several beneficial properties, including antibacterial and antioxidant properties, and a relaxant effect.

These clever research nurses devised a simple plan: Get their patients to consume *a liter of water*, or about four cups, by the end of the breakfast hour. By extending the breakfast social time, residents drank more. The nurses in effect preloaded and soaked those in their care early in the day, and we recommend the same in the Quench Plan (see chapter 8).

With this important strategy they were able to correlate reduced paramedic interventions and intercept hospital admissions.[15]

Quince

Quince is legendary as a hydrating fruit. Its pastelike, gel-like consistency has been cultivated all over the world, from its origins in Turkey, through the Iberian peninsula, to England by the 1300s, and on to the New World. In Chile, traditional village women, caring for their elder parents, would use a daily dose of sweetened quince paste to keep the elders happy while they attended to younger children. This paste was formed into oblong medallions to rest and dissolve on the tongue, and further, these medallions were also the last food given to ease the passage of death. Paste presses or small wooden pestles were carved with exquisite good-bye wishes or blessings and then embossed into the medallions. Versions of this practice continue, and quince jam is still offered in Argentina during hospice care for hydration when drinking is difficult.

We are surrounded by people we love—let's make sure they stay hydrated and healthy, too! We'll show how you can help properly hydrate them in our Quench Plan.

CHAPTER 7

Antiaging, the Skin, and Beauty

I will do water—beautiful, blue water.

—*Claude Monet*

We hate the word *anti-aging*. Because aging is exactly what we *want* to do. Aging is actually becoming more and more of who we are. It is about the constant growth, addition, and development that leads us to new levels of wisdom and determines our very capacity for handling life. You naturally accumulate, over time, experience; life stories; knocks and celebrations; and, above all, the wisdom they contain. We relish what those lessons taught us and how we've learned from them. That's called aging, so let's champion it. The real question is not how to anti-age, but to *age well*. The simple answer is not to dry out.

The ability to remain a vital person as we age, full of energy, alert, and buoyant is all we have been discussing throughout this book. How could hydration not have a rejuvenating impact on aging? Recall watering that wilted plant. The new science of hydration equates water intake with energy intake. In *Quench* we have given you the science of why that is so. Hydration is our most potent and best pathway to, well, we are not going to say anti-aging, but instead, life *expectancy*, the kind that is full of energy. The life expectancy we all want is vibrating with alertness, being aware and experiencing the exquisite and connected network your body is. Our inner water orchestrates the elements within us. That's beauty!

If hydration is not already inside of you, then all those beauty creams, moisturizers, serums, and capsules are not holding in very much. Those products are important, but the most important part of their job is to support the hydration already within you. Every esthetician knows hydration and good skin start from within, and great estheticians make hydration their first recommendation. Water and wisdom go together.

HYDRATION AND SKIN

Skin is the largest organ of the body, protecting our other precious organs from assaults from environment and, most important for our purposes, holding in our water. And while you may think of skin as playing defense, its foremost job is actually playing offense, tossing out unwanted materials through pores. We don't usually think of skin this way, but that's just how our pores work. That is why skin is a major hydration organ: both holding hydration in and taking out the trash, too. Outgoing flow is as important as incoming drinking. The skin has roughly one thousand pores per square inch, through which we perspire.

The pore function of the skin could use some help staying effective, and the best help it can get is induced sweating. Before, we have talked about sweat in sports mostly as a cooling mechanism. But here we are talking about sweat therapeutically, not solely for skin health but for whole body hydration. So let's get on to sweat.

SWEATING FOR BEAUTY, THE OUTFLOW OF HYDRATION

Sweat transforms waste in the body from an oil- or a lipid-soluble chemical into a water-soluble chemical, then flushes it out through the pores. The task of the skin in hydration is as central as fascia, blood circulation, or lymph circulation. Dr. Stephen Genuis from the University of Alberta has published a few studies that establish sweat as a waste-removal system. Specifically sweating can increase removal of heavy metals, such as mercury, lead, and cadmium, and some chemical toxicants like bisphenol A and phthalates.[1] Sweat may have antimicrobial properties, in that its pH may prevent the bacteria from living in your pores and causing acne. Mild to moderate sweating also opens pores and allows the release of clogging oils and dirt. It is important, though, to clean your skin immediately after sweating so the dirt and toxins in the sweat don't get reabsorbed into your skin. Skin needs our attention and renewal both from the inside and the outside. We can now understand that inside-and-outside skin care is a cooperative venture.

DR. DANA'S CASE STUDY

Irene

"Dr. Dana, I need to look good for my first day at school!"

Irene, an eighteen-year-old student, had come in with her mom, also a patient of mine, for a checkup. She was a straight-A student and would attend an Ivy League college in the fall. Like a typical teenager, she was very conscious of how she looked, and she had been battling acne and her weight. She was anxious to get help before she set off to school. Her anxiety may have caused her irritable bowel syndrome; she had a lot of stomachaches, and she alternated between constipation and diarrhea. The stomachaches were nothing new—her mom told me she'd had them as child, and she had been colicky as a baby.

I first asked about her diet.

"I'm a vegetarian." When I pressed her on her diet, I found out she ate a lot of pasta, bread, cheese, and dairy.

Knowing that dairy can cause inflammation and stomach issues, I asked her to eliminate it for three weeks. I gave her a list of dairy substitutes and asked her to swap in whole grains, like quinoa or brown rice, for the simple carbs she was eating. I also asked her to eat fish to up her omega-3 levels, which I suspected were low, but I had to wait for lab results to confirm. To my delight, she was willing to include fish, because she really wanted clear skin. I gave her some easy fish ideas to try, like a mild white fish (such as Dover sole); she remembered being a fan of shrimp and other shellfish, as well, so she promised she would mix it up. I also put her on the Quench five-day program.

When she came back two weeks later, her skin was remarkably improved, not a pimple popping up, and she was moving her bowels regularly, without any pain. She was ecstatic to be looking and feeling so good after feeling bad for so long. Her blood work had come back all normal, except in her fatty acid profile. Her omega-3s were low, just as I had suspected, but she had been good about increasing her fish intake, and she had even added salmon to her menu.

We were so pleased with her results, but the question that immediately popped up for us was: How is she going to continue this at school? We talked thoroughly about how to handle the impending school year. Committed to her health, she asked the university's housing department if she could have a blender and small fridge in her room. She also inquired about locations for farmers' markets near her school, and of course she had a handy printout of the Quench Plan with her. She remains happy and healthy; her skin is just beautiful, and she continues to get straight As.

The Anthropology of Sauna

Every culture around the world has a sweat strategy for cleansing, renewing, and rejuvenating, through releasing hydration. Ancient Asia Minor developed the famous steam-based Turkish baths; the ancient Romans built their "thermae" at the center of civic life, the Russians had their relaxing "banya." Traditional Japanese raised hot bathing and sweating to the highest level of health care and body beauty with the "onsen." And saunas in indigenous cultures were a must, a gathering place for health and elevation through communal sacred events. The Native Americans used their sweat lodges; the Lenapes on Manhattan Island made their sweat lodges from the lasting wood of the tulip tree, whose inner bark released a healing resin in the steam. The Incas used flora medicinal baths as part of their sweat traditions. However, one of the most clinically studied forms of health through sweating is the famous Finnish sauna. Dr. Rhonda Patrick, a biomedical scientist and founder of the FoundMyFitness.com website, is an expert on sauna effects on health, recently reported that the positive effects of heat on our systems comes from stimulating heat shock proteins inside our cells.[2] In addition, cold plunges after hot saunas are also widely recorded by cultures in northern climates, which acclimated people to their winter environments. Getting outside our "comfort zones" indeed brings resiliency on the cellular level.

INFRARED SAUNAS AND INFRARED LIGHT

There are volumes written on hydration and skin care, but we are going bring the new science of water molecules to the discussion.

Using infrared lamps on your skin has real, clinically established hydrating effects. This makes sense if, indeed, light waves promote gel water in our bodies. As we talked about earlier, Dr. Pollack's work has shown that infrared light is the most powerful producer of EZ water. The more infrared, the more gel water. We should see measurable improvement in skin appearance. Improvement from simple infrared bulbs can be measured and were: In a 2014 study, Alexander Wunsch and his team treated people with infrared light, and their patients experienced significantly improved skin complexion. This German study took very precise measurements both above and below the skin and used ultrasound to measure collagen density. The test confirmed not only significant improvement in the skin itself but a measurable increase in intradermal collagen. And they also verified the safety of skin rejuvenation from infrared. These effects came simply from sitting under light.[3]

For us, that means rejuvenated skin simply using light and water. We have been eternally searching for the fountain of youth. Could it be water plus light?

DR. DANA'S CASE STUDY

Denise

Denise, a forty-five-year-old yoga instructor, is extremely healthy and eats a great plant-based diet. She came in my office to be treated for Hashimoto's disease, a thyroid condition she has had since her twenties. She had always been careful about keeping that condition in check, and she commented that she felt healthy and had no complaints, as always. Although Denise wasn't a typical candidate for the plan, I decided to put her on the Quench program, as I suspected she wasn't optimally hydrated—most people aren't—and see if we could elicit an even better health profile.

After a few weeks, she e-mailed me to let me know how she was doing. She couldn't believe how much better she felt since getting more liquids in her: "My skin is radiant!" She realized that she probably was just not drinking enough water during the day. "How innocuous hydration seems," she wrote, "but the incredible results by changing my habits just slightly are mind-boggling." She ended her e-mail by saying that since being more hydrated, her yoga practice has become "off the chain." And of course, she let her students know what she has learned. What a way to pay it forward!

THE BEAUTY OF SLEEP

Beauty and sleep are connected—you have heard the phrase "Get your beauty rest" a million times, right? There is a new reason behind this adage, and it's detoxification. Dr. Maiken Nedergaard and her colleagues at the University of Rochester Medical Center stunned scientists by discovering an entire drainage system hidden in specialized brain cells.[4] This system operates similarly to the lymph system, but drains waste products solely from the brain. They call it the glymphatic system. This is a major new discovery. And it works at night, during sleep, creating an increase in flow by *60 percent*, like the nighttime sanitation crew. It's as if our brains, once free from "thought traffic," use this perfect time to flush away debris. Nedergaard says, "Understanding precisely how and when the brain activates the glymphatic system and clears waste is a critical first step in efforts to potentially make it work more efficiently." All this flow and circulation depends on adequate hydration levels. Who knew that lying flat, closing our eyes, and drifting off was part of our hydration story?

MASSAGE

There has never been a moment in human history where massage has not been used among human populations. Massage therapy is older than recorded time. Massage is even used by primates. There is, of course, a great variety of traditions. So many cultures around the globe practiced end-of-day massage, either on themselves or on one another. It was the reward for the work of the day. We should not forsake this ancient health practice.

Why Massages Hydrate

All-around massage is foremost about moving fluids in the body. We have long known that massage moves blood through the circulation system, but new research on fascia shows that massage moves hydration as well. Recall the work of Dr. Jean-Claude Guimberteau, whose video was introduced in chapter 3 recorded water droplets moving along the fascia network. Hands-on massage pulses hydration through the fascia, as well as the blood and the lymph system, so massage affects a number of systems at once. Specialized massages, like lymph or facial massage, literally move waste down the line for quicker exit.

Benefits of Massage

We know empirically that massage has therapeutic benefit. It is a $6 billion industry, which speak volumes for its benefits. It has been shown to improve immunity in breast cancer patients; even Memorial Sloan Kettering Cancer Center offers it as part of their cancer therapy. However, there are remarkably very few formal studies on massage therapy in the medical journals.

Ask anyone who has had a massage; the benefits are clear to them. Their skin is glowing, their pain is lessened, their anger and anxiety are reduced, and their energy is improved. So many things happen to your system when you get a massage. Besides the all-body-fluid movement, your collagen proteins are being stimulated to produce more, your relaxation response kicks in (but you knew that), kinks are being removed, and deep breathing probably occurs!

Self-Massage

You don't have to use professional massage therapists; self-massage works, too. You can apply pressure, moving liquid and stretching tissue, firing up those cells to go off and do some work to keep you optimal. Now you have new motivation to rub down your legs while you watch TV. What is great about self-massage is the giveback to your underappreciated body. "You can take time to sit down and be just focused on yourself," says Masae Shimomoto, a massage therapist at Complete Wellness in New York City. To begin a self-massage practice, she recommends you start simply with your fingers, hands, and feet. Variations of such self-massage are found throughout Asia, and all are ancient techniques. Quench plan users noticed they had started

giving themselves massages far more often. One to practice during the workday is working over hands and fingers.

Movement as a Form of Self-Massage

From reading about how fascia works and cells fire, you could
recast all movement now as a form of self-massage, or cellular
massage, whether you do your own hands-on from the outside
or through self-stretch generating movement from the inside.
Self-stretch throughout the day brings new levels of fluidity but
also new levels of brain function, cell function, and whole body
vitality. Did we mention hydration?

Brushing Up on Ancient Skin Care

Dry brushing is as old as our ancestors. Rubbing down the skin with
leaves, flowers, mashed sticks (which is really just an early iteration
of a brush), seaweeds, sand, clays, pebbles, and fabrics have been
natural forms of skin health since we could walk erect with hands
free. These techniques exist in all cultures and are often associated
with ritual and renewal, rightly so. From our new perspective we
can say rubbing the body works on many levels, stimulating skin
collagen growth, exfoliating the old skin, uncovering new cells,
moving fluids, and speeding waste materials out. In the shower,
before you turn on the tap, is the perfect time to dry-brush.

Massage Your Face

We may worry that massaging and stretching our skin on our
face may age it or loosen it prematurely, but we are learning

quite the opposite. Cells make collagen under pressure, and collagen is the underlying structure of skin. Touch literally renews. There are fascinating approaches to massaging your face that come out of very old traditions with great results.

Tonya Zavasta, author of *Beautiful on Raw* and a skin and aging expert, updates the old Russian traditions on face massage and skin care by recommending that you actually dry-brush your face, a novel idea to many of us. She warns that if you do it, however, use a softer brush than one typically uses in dry body brushing, and brush in small circles.

In the Hindi tradition, they do not dry-brush the face but massage the face with oils, while also practicing forms of acupressure and tapping on the face.

From the qi gong tradition, famed for beauty of movement leading to endurance and long life expectancy, large groups of elders in China participate first thing every morning in parks all over the country. Less known is that they are also geniuses at facial massage, which is considered just a natural extension of full body movement. They simply rub their faces and necks briskly with the backs of their hands and would never go a day without doing so.

Why Posture Is an Act of Beauty and a Form of Micromassage

When you stand in good alignment, you are actually activating a whole series of micromovements. Good posture is a dynamic act. Rethink posture as standing dynamically with tiny concentrated yet relaxed movements, just like a swing bridge swaying in the wind. This equilibrium concept is a truly new understanding of posture that further links it to hydration through adjusting micromovement. Not only does good posture increase the flow of liquid through both our fascia tissues and our blood circulation, it also opens up our lungs for deeper breathing and takes pressure off our whole digestive system. Check in with your spine and posture throughout the day. If you are scrunched over, be aware of it and fix it with our following micromovements.

Dr. Daniel Fenster is the clinic director of Complete Wellness, a clinician for more than thirty years, and the author of a forthcoming book on posture. He states, "Everyone knows posture is important—our mothers told us so! But why is posture important? And why is it important for hydration? When there is good posture, also known as proper alignment, everything in the body functions better. Additionally, less stress is put on the musculature to better retain normal hydration." He agrees with us that this modern-day problem of hunching over our desks at work and all that texting are dehydrating us because the body gets out of alignment.

Another posture expert, Dr. Guy Voyer, DO, originator of the ELDOA Method of fascial therapy, also traces how important spinal alignment is to hydration. Without alignment, he says, the spinal "disc loses its water content (dehydrates) and loses its hydrostatic pressure (osmotic pressure)." Simply put, even if we were well hydrated, without osmotic pressure, it is more difficult to get fluid where we need it. Therefore dynamic posture is a very important hydration strategy.

But we can reestablish, through posture, our own optimal hydration. Dr. Adalbert I. Kapandji, a renowned orthopedic surgeon, says, "For every inch of forward head posture, the weight of the head on the spine increases by an additional 10 pounds."[5] Not only are we carrying a heavier head by leaning forward, we are significantly constricting the passage of synovial fluid to our brain, and down goes its function.

Posture Flow

Social psychologist Amy Cuddy's 2012 viral TED Talk, "Your Body Language May Shape Who You Are," used science to change many minds about how posture affects us and those who see us. In her talk she explained her experiment to find out if "power postures" lowered stress chemicals. She had tested students' saliva to find out if standing for two minutes in certain poses with a sense of power reduced, among other chemicals, cortisol. In two minutes, cortisol dropped between 15 and 25 percent. So posture change alone led to chemical changes that configured your brain to be more confident and comfortable.[6]

Posture, on many levels, then, becomes a hydrating strategy, not just something to please your mom. Here is a visual aid to help you think about where your head aligns in relation to your spine: Imagine your head as if it were a balloon tied on the end of stick, bobbing freely. That is a good picture to begin with. Elongating or stretching up the space between your hips and ribs will also get you into good posture, and by the way, it will shrink your waistline, too.

From an anthropological point of view, our perception of beauty includes how we stand. Women and men who stand up straight are seen as more attractive around the world and are perceived as leaders.

For getting to posture perfect quickly, we are fans of the Egoscue Method, developed by Pete Egoscue in the 1970s. His posture therapy offers a thorough and very short routine to retrain your awareness. We love it because this technique understands the relationship between hydration and drainage of the lymph system, and it is one of the only posture programs that has you simply lying on your back with your feet up on a chair. Our kind of exercise! You can innovate with pillows to do it in bed at night while you read. And add a few micromovements while you are at it.

POSTURE IS WALKING MICROMOVEMENT

Now that we have talked about standing straight, how about taking it on the road? The best place to install good posture is by walking. Walking with aligned posture is a dynamic activity, not a onetime, breath-held-in event. Another fast way to great posture comes from Teresa Tapp, founder of T-Tapp and author of *Fit and Fabulous in Fifteen Minutes*. Early on in her career she realized that small movements do ten times the work. She also realized we were all trying to get to good posture from the wrong spot. "Don't throw out your chest," she implores. "Lift your ribs, and you will immediately feel you back muscles engage." Those back muscles are made to support your spine while walking.

In addition, Mary Bond, the author of *The New Rules of Posture: How to Sit, Stand, and Move in the Modern World*, connects posture with improved cognitive function, heightening our alertness and focus. Since this kind of dynamic good posture moves out waste materials in our system naturally, how could it not affect our thinking for the better?

300 Moves

Esther Gokhale is well-known for investigating posture from an anthropological standpoint. She has looked at traditions across the world of people and goes back to how babies balance. Anatomically, we are capable of more than three hundred different kinds of movement, yet in our modern culture, by the time we reach adulthood, we are down to a range of about thirty. That really is surprising, and it also leads to pain. Especially lower back pain. In Gokhale's book, *8 Steps to a Pain-Free Back*, she takes on the challenge of the limited range modern living has required of us and helps reverse the cost of our desks, cars, and generally immobile living.

WHY MEDITATION IS HYDRATING

Dr. Roger Jahnke, founder of the Institute of Integral Qigong and Tai Chi and author of the influential book *The Healer Within*, has been a tireless advocate for bringing health and stress-management strategies from the East to the West. He speaks of the ancient Asian techniques that interrupt the stress signals, those stress neurochemicals and hormones that dehydrate us. Remembering to drop our stress and tension many times a day changes our biochemistry by altering our neurotransmitters. Don't wait until you get home to unload but practice micro-meditations in the same way, or even at the same time, as micro-movements. Chin circles or head rolls are great ways to move into a short meditation. Taking care to consciously dump stress and tension as you go through your day will get you out from under the accumulated burden on your body. Sloughing off a little here and there, maybe while you're sipping something, makes sense.

We live in a highly sustained stress culture—no one escapes the stop-and-go traffic, the unreasonable deadlines, the interruptions, the online passwords, and other accumulating irritations of modern life. When we are stressed, our levels of cortisol and other stress hormones go up. And you know what? Those hormones are found in all fluids inside you—and can be measured in our blood and saliva. And those hormones, over time, can do damage to our body, like increased blood pressure, weight gain, and lower immune function. But you can dilute those chemicals with powerful hydration. Seriously. Remember you are 99 percent water by molecular count, so don't "soak" yourself in worry. Instead, use water and meditation to dilute those stress chemicals. Here we offer two meditations to break the loop of stress.

SINKING AWAY

Back to Dr. Roger Jahnke, an extraordinary visionary for merging Eastern and Western approaches to health. He is also a leader in bringing antistress techniques into hospitals and communities around the world. His book *The Healer Within* merges movement with meditation. We have included our twist on Dr. Jahnke's "Remembering Breath" meditation here, with our own "water" twist at the end to make it a hydrating experience, too.

While sitting or standing, straighten up to your best comfort. Bring your head up and your chin in enough to feel your spinal cord aligning right up and into the back of your skull, like someone is pulling you up by a string. Draw a deep breath, which you will be much more able to do now that your lungs are freed up from all that scrunching we do. Close your eyes and imagine yourself standing in a pool, a lake, or an ocean of water up to your chest or neck. As you draw in that single breath, imagine slipping slowly under the surface. Imagine the world sliding away as you sink, just you and your breath and the cool silence. You can release your breath however you want.

This meditation can be as short as the one deep breath, or you can practice "disappearing" throughout your day as you transition from one task to the next. This simple one-breath sequence breaks the loop of worry and returns your autonomic system to restart. It is amazing what one breath can do, though you may find you want to stay down "there" longer. Recall that deep breathing brings vapor hydration into your lungs.

BEAUTY WATER

If you are in the habit of carrying a water bottle, we want to make that water bottle more hydrating. Beauty water recipes are designed to be simple and require no blending, bringing more gel water into your average water bottle. Any plant can assist in helping your water get more gel in it. Adding berries, citrus fruit, cucumbers, sprigs of herbs, or other flavorings to your water makes it easier to consume the water you need to keep yourself hydrated.

We suggest you try each single ingredient by itself in water to better discover which flavors you prefer, before pairing them with other flavors. Then you can mix and match. Add any one of the following ingredients to 16 ounces of water. Stir well.

- ½ teaspoon pomegranate powder or 1 teaspoon liquid pomegranate concentrate
- 1 teaspoon rose petal jam
- 1 teaspoon honey, plus a sprig of basil, rosemary, or thyme
- 10 goji berries
- 10 fresh or frozen blueberries, raspberries, or other berries
- 1 splash balsamic vinegar to water with berries
- ½ teaspoon ground turmeric and 1 teaspoon maple syrup
- ½- to 1-inch piece ginger, depending on taste, diced
- ½ teaspoon beet root powder

Pomegranate Beauty Water

Pomegranates are loaded with powerful antioxidants, vitamins, and minerals. Moreover, the oil from the seeds has been shown to have anti-inflammatory benefits, and it increases collagen in the skin.[7]

2 tablespoons pomegranate seeds
⅛ teaspoon coarse sea salt
3½ cups filtered or spring water

In a 1-quart, wide-mouth canning jar, coarsely crush the pomegranate seeds with the back of a wooden spoon. Add the salt and water over the seeds. This can be refrigerated or enjoyed at room temperature, and there's no need to strain.

There is no topical cream that can match inner hydration. In the next chapter, our Quench Plan will get you on your way to looking vital while adding to what you expect out of life.

CHAPTER 8

The Quench Plan

Under any circumstance, simply do your best, and you will avoid self-judgment, self-abuse and regret.

—*Don Miguel Ruiz*

Hydration is the most potent intervention you can do for yourself because by molecular count, you are 99 percent water. Do you want to feel more focused at work? Do you want more energy to make it through the day without that afternoon slump? Do you want to walk out of your work day *and* still have energy for your evening?

The Quench Plan will get you to a new level of hydration, healing, and energy with easy-to-follow instructions for the smartest drinking. Recall our essential three principles of hydration we have laid out for you in the previous chapters:

1. **Absorption:** Get the maximum absorption from the water you drink so it gets to the cellular level, where it can produce energy and not just pass through.

2. **Water from Food:** Eating foods high in water content can boost deep hydration—our plant-rich smoothies, for

instance, will hydrate you far better than the same amount of bottled water and deliver high-level nutrition to boot.

3. **Movement:** We'll show you easy-to-do yet crucial micromovements to deliver hydration right to key places like neck and joints to keep you flexible and pain free.

How can you get more hydration into your day? Well it's easy:

1. Sip a "smart smoothie." It packs more hydrating power in a glass than water.
2. Add a few drinks at key points of the day.
3. Eat foods that hydrate vs. dehydrate.

We designed the five-day Quench Plan to get your hydration up—this isn't a plan to lose weight or inches, although you very well may. And this isn't about counting calories; this is about finally getting to optimal hydration. It's a plan to get your entire system what it needs to function optimally. You will feel better, sleep better, move better, even age better. Cognition and physical performance improve, as well as skin, digestion, and ease of movement. And don't be surprised if you lose a few pounds. But that number on the scale isn't as important as how you feel. This five-day plan shows you how to start, but your long-term practice is sure to balance your weight and improve your health on every front. To make it easy, we have designed Quench to simply add a few small, new things. We designed these small practices to ignite long-term shifts in your energy and health.

Why five days? It's the window of a typical workweek, so it's something you can easily add to your routine. And by day five, you really begin to notice a difference. When you see the results, you'll want to keep Quenching. And if you fall off the "water wagon," as all of us do, you'll know and have your recovery plan ready to go. Return to your inspiring Quench plan.

Here we offer clear, simple, and easy instructions, recipes, and tips that lead you through the five full days to get you to somewhere truly new and needed in our modern environments. Water is fuel, and we show you where and how to "fuel up" for higher levels of energy and focus. We've given you a choice of one or two smoothies per day, optimal timing for drinking, instructions for daily movements, and examples of healthy and hydrating eating. That's it.

We keep your taste buds happy in our five-day plan by adding a new ingredient every day. Use our second recipe provided each day if you're feeling bored. Your choice: Either keep it simple for five days with the daily recipe, or try an entirely new one from our recipe section for each of the five days. All optimally hydrate. Mix and match during the five days and into your future.

What is great about our Quench design is its gentleness. Remember, hydration is the baseline of all homeostasis or equilibrium in the body, and that is what we are doing with the five-day plan: recalibrating your hydration levels. We don't have to warn you against possible headaches, detox reactions, rash outbreaks, constipation, or hunger you have to push through. Hydration does nothing but good for you, advancing you back to buoyancy.

SMOOTHIES SAVE THE DAY

The heart of the program are the tasty smoothies. If there is only one thing you do to change your hydration intake, add a smoothie to your diet every day. That alone will be doing a great service to your body, hydration packaged with dense nutrition and fiber. We provide you with several delicious recipes, but feel free to create your own. We also suggest healthy meal ideas to promote proper hydration from your plate as well as in your glass. After you eat and drink, we show you how to deliver that hydration all the way to your tissues through simple but effective micromovements and breathing techniques. This whole approach works in unison to increase your body's fluidity through hydration, nutrition, flexibility, and mind-body integration.

Why are smoothies the foundation of the Quench Plan? Smoothies offer the perfect combination of nutrition and hydration. They not only amplify hydration through providing the water locked in plants, but according to Dr. Joel Fuhrman, president of the Nutritional Research Foundation, chewing food releases only about 35 percent of the nutritional materials in that food. And according to Fuhrman, blending our food makes those nutrients up to *90 percent* bioavailable—meaning they are more easily absorbed.

How would you like to increase your nutrition intake without purchasing expensive supplements, without having to eat an extra ton of food, and while taking care of your hydration needs at the same time? In our stressed life we are not even really chewing our food, we are gulping it! Even with a great organic salad, unless you are really chewing that forkful into liquid, you aren't breaking down the food particles enough to fully extract all the nutrients to be had. This means more than half the value of your expensive salad is being wasted. Great news then, that blending does that chewing brilliantly for us. And if you keep your first couple of sips of smoothies on your tongue for a few seconds before you swallow, you start the whole process by triggering your body's own digestive enzymes produced when you salivate.

Smoothies also provide fiber that efficiently slows down the passage of hydration and nutrition, allowing a longer transit time for nutrients and liquids to be truly absorbed. This is one of our main findings. Drinking too much bottled water too quickly can flash-flood your system unless it is accompanied with those food fibers to aid absorption. All that drinking can actually flush out the very important electrolytes and nutrients that metabolize and accomplish full hydration. Absorption can also save you from too many visits to the bathroom. Smoothies can help slow down the passage of fluids so your system will actually have time to absorb. And smoothies can virtually eliminate the dreaded constipation: your food starts its journey already hydrated.

DR. DANA'S CASE STUDY

Danielle

Several years ago, Danielle, forty-nine at the time, first started seeing me for menopausal weight gain and exhaustion. She kept gaining and losing the same five pounds. "It's like a yo-yo; every time I think I am getting ahead, I step on the scale and feel defeated." Complicating matters, she was prediabetic and had a sluggish thyroid. I put her on thyroid medication, HRT, and a medication for her blood sugar called Metformin. She did well, losing the weight that had dogged her. Recently, she came in for a checkup—she was still keeping the pounds off, but she did complain of a little constipation. She had been on a trendy diet, the Whole 30, a strict program of whole foods and no grains.

It was around the time that we had been asking some of my patients to take part in an early informal study, testing out the five-day Quench program. She was on board, but then I never heard from her. Until the day we delivered this very book to our publisher.

That day was also Gina's birthday, and she decided to celebrate both her birthday and turning in the *Quench* manuscript with a solo glass of wine at a bar before meeting her family for dinner. At the random bar she slipped into, a woman sat down next to Gina and they started chatting. The conversation turned to medicine, and the woman revealed that she saw a wonderful holistic doctor. And that doctor was writing a book on hydration. Gina's jaw dropped, and she asked, "Is it Dr. Dana Cohen?"

"Yes! Do you know her?" the woman, who turned out to be Danielle, replied.

"Not only do I know her, I am writing that book with her!"

"Oh my gosh, I did the program and I feel fantastic!"

How likely is this encounter? Danielle turned out to be one of the very first Quench practitioners, rediscovered on the day we finished writing.

Since Danielle had felt bad about not returning the survey, she followed up, calling Dana the following week. She reported that she had been suffering with headaches all summer, but by the *second* morning on the program, her headaches were gone. She also said she had more energy and was very much awake and focused at work. She noticed, too, that by the fourth day, the bags under her eyes were much smaller.

She continues to follow the Whole 30 diet, but she has incorporated more hydrating fruits and veggies, and she loves doing her micromovements every morning to start her day.

As you begin with our simple smoothie foundational base recipe, you will discover yourself wanting to add new ingredients and making up your own variations. Remember the simple principle that leafy greens are 98 percent water and full of nutrition to boot. This will motivate you to find ways to include your own workable, likable variations of leafy greens in your smoothies, which make all vegetables taste flavorful, variable, and delicious.

You will develop a sense for what pleases you, for example, how thin or thick you like your smoothies. You'll learn by practice your preference for combinations and texture, even discovering that blending for one minute gives you a different-tasting smoothie than blending for two minutes. Various brands of blenders differ in how long they need to blend for a smoothness you like.

We believe a boot camp–style approach is unsustainable. Instead, think of a compass where one small change in degree takes you to an entirely new destination. All we ask is you try it for five days—you'll be on your way to becoming more hydrated on a deeper level. In those five days you will feel energetic, lighter, and less stiff and have better mood and focus. And while we designed the five-day Quench Plan to get you to the next level of hydration, we believe that you will want to use these techniques for a lifelong practice. We have given you all you need so that you can continue to customize and refine to your own changing needs.

After you start, you will want to continue on your hydration journey. While this plan is designed to kick-start your health, once you see how good you feel, you will want to use these techniques forever.

The Elderly and Smoothies

Remember Gina's attempts to address her mother's chronic dehydration, outlined in the preface? To remedy her mother's issue, Gina added ground chia seeds to her mother's morning orange juice. That was the end to her mom's frequent urinary tract infections. Why grind the seeds? Grinding releases more gel by exposing more surface area, and the powder doesn't irritate the digestive tract. For those who worry about seeds and diverticulitis, a condition so often present in the dehydrated elderly, there's no cause for concern on that front. The seeds are pulverized, and there's no chance of them getting stuck in the outpockets of diverticulosis. We care about our elders and especially hope they will use the program, however much they can practically implement it. If making smoothies isn't viable for an elder, switch to green or red powders and add in the ground chia seeds. Beyond that, just toss ground chia seeds in a glass of juice, as Gina did for her mother. Our elderly needn't be thirsty.[1] And this *is* a perfect plan for the elderly: with plant foods' more absorptive power, constipation will be reduced through higher fiber, and nutritive vitamins and minerals will help with brain brightness and strength, among other things. Add easy and gentle micromovements to help with agility and balance, even if you are in a wheelchair or bed bound.

THE UPSIDE TO PEEING

Hydration is not only about intake; it's also about about output. In the Quench Plan, there is a good amount of water going into your system throughout the day. You may experience more frequent urination. We have news for you: This isn't a downside.

We are all supposed to be peeing every two to three hours. It's just a great sign that you are well hydrated. More waste is going out more quickly, and this gets you moving—just think, all that walking to the bathroom is good daily movement! If you're well hydrated, you should be urinating six to seven times a day. How many times have you gone the whole day at work and noticed you haven't used the bathroom even once? We are here to tell you that is not good. When you feel the results of less fatigue, you will welcome those bathroom breaks.

As your body water mass finds its own optimal level, your whole system should feel so much better. Take notice of the ways in which you experience improvements. Look for less headaches, more energy, more flexibility, brighter mood, clearer skin, less bloating, and better sleep. *Celebrate those signs.*

This plan is great for almost anyone. If you have any underlying health issues, like diabetes and heart conditions, then you should consult your doctor or nutritionist. They could help tailor the meal suggestions that fit your condition. Read through the plan first to see what delights are ahead of you.

HOW TO GET STARTED ON THE FIVE-DAY QUENCH PLAN

Equipment you will need:

- Blender of any kind (see Blenders 101 in chapter 9)
- Water bottle, minimum 16 ounces, preferably glass or stainless steel and dishwasher safe.

Shopping list for the five-day plans (both cold and hot ingredients, select as you please):

- Alfalfa sprouts (1 package)
- Apple cider vinegar, raw (16 ounces)
- Butter, grass-fed, unsalted (1 stick) or ghee (1 container)
- Cardamom or cinnamon, ground (1 container)
- Cashews or raw nuts or ground seeds, like sunflower, pumpkin, hemp (1 package)
- Chia seeds (8-ounce package)—ground is best for absorption; grind them in a coffee grinder, or use them whole.
- Coconut milk, unsweetened (1 can, full fat, for savings, or 1 carton for ease)
- Coconut water, unsweetened (two 8-ounce containers), optional
- Cucumbers (3)
- Ginger root (2-to-4-inch piece)
- Honey, raw (1 jar)
- Lemons (2)
- Limes (2)
- Maple syrup or stevia (1 small bottle)
- Pear (1) or apple (1)
- Pomegranate juice concentrate (1 bottle). Substitute with grape, blueberry, or cherry juice concentrates. If you can't find concentrates, use pomegranate juice or substitute orange or grapefruit juice (1 carton)
- Raspberries, frozen or fresh (1 container)
- Salt, natural unrefined sea or rock (finely ground)
- Tea, chamomile and/or licorice (5 tea bags)
- Water, filtered or spring, distilled in a pinch but be sure to add salt as directed (2 gallons); see What Are the Differences Between All the Different Waters?

What Are the Differences Between All the Different Waters?

Purified water is defined by the lack of contaminants in it. It is a legal term, and in order to be labeled as such, it must contain extremely low levels of impurities. It is usually produced by some type of distillation process where the water is boiled and its steam is captured and used to produce **distilled** water. Other ways to purify is reverse osmosis and deionization. Unfortunately, minerals and electrolytes are also removed.

Spring water flows naturally from an underground source (an aquifer) that is filtered by the earth itself and is rich in earth's minerals, although it may not meet the legal definition of purified water. Spring water is best if you go and collect it yourself directly from the source. Bottled "spring" water isn't much better than tap water. That water "straight from the spring" being sold to you by large bottling companies is typically transported back to their bottling centers by big diesel trucks and is chlorinated to protect it from bacteria. Not really the image you were thinking of.

Mineral water comes from a protected underground source and must contain some minerals, typically magnesium and sulfur compounds. Mineral water also has natural gases and is effervescent in nature.

Artesian water is drawn from a well that taps a confined aquifer containing groundwater under positive pressure.

Seltzer, sparkling water, and **club sodas** are basically bubbly water made by the process of carbonation—or adding carbon dioxide. While we prefer natural sparkling mineral water, these are fine to drink and basically the same as water. The only downside we can think of is it may upset your stomach or worsen your reflux; then it's obviously not a good idea. And stay away from the ones that have added sweeteners or, worse, added artificial sweeteners.

WHY OUR SHOPPING LIST IS SO HYDRATING

Our shopping list is made up of foods that (1) help absorb hydration and (2) activate the charge of water molecules. We list here why each food offers specific hydration support, although these foods offer other nutrition as well.

Alfalfa sprouts: Alfalfa is more than 90 percent water and full of valuable trace minerals, such as manganese, vital for efficient digestion. Apart from the high mineral content, which activates the battery-like charge in collaboration with alfalfa's high water content, it is also a rich source of vitamins A, B, C, E, and K.

Apple cider vinegar, raw: Apple cider vinegar is, of course, a liquid, but it is also potassium rich, drawing water through to the inside of the cell. It is also alkalizing, and that speeds digestion and may help lower your blood sugar. We recommend using raw apple cider vinegar (ACV) throughout the Quench Plan. ACV is produced from aged apples' sugars through yeast fermentation. The raw form, usually cloudy in appearance, contains many vitamins, minerals, proteins, friendly bacteria, and enzymes. Minerals especially are required for hydration to reach all the way into tissues and cells. When it is pasteurized, it loses much of the health benefits to which raw apple cider vinegar has been linked. Raw ACV has been shown to improve insulin sensitivity and lower blood sugars in humans. And in some animal studies, it can lower cholesterol and triglyceride levels.

Butter, grass-fed: Butter may seem an unusual food for hydration, but we are watching the emerging science showing fats, as lipids, have an important role to play in transferring water outside the cell to the inside of the cell.

Cardamom: Cardamom has diuretic properties, to release bloat and clean out the urinary tract, bladder, and kidneys, removing waste, salt, excess water, and toxins. Cardamom can help combat infections, too.

Cashews: Cashews have the hydrating combination of high mineral content, like copper, phosphorus, zinc, magnesium, iron, and notably selenium, an uncommon but essential mineral. Cashews also contain a lot of those heart-healthy monounsaturated fats.

Chia: Chia is the highest gel-releasing seed and is very rich in healthy omega-3 fatty acids. Fatty acids are necessary to move water into the cell. Chia seeds, with all their nutrient density, also lay down a protective, permeable film all along your digestive tract, protecting you from acids and spicy foods, allowing in only good stuff. Chia slows the release of insulin, lowers blood pressure, and makes gentle, regular elimination inevitable. Chia also has ten grams of fiber per ounce, which retains hydration for long-lasting use. Chia is an easily digestible source of protein, about four grams per ounce. A true superfood!

Cinnamon: High in antioxidants and anti-inflammatory agents, we use it to counteract any sugar issues in our recipes, as cinnamon is known to regulate blood glucose levels.

Coconut milk: Coconuts carry great nutrition and taste delicious. The milk is high in those very fats that help regulate water flow into the cell. Coconuts offer far better hydration than almond or soy milk.

Coconut water: Coconut water is very rich in electrolytes, which are minerals activated with electrical charge, and provide energy to our cells.

Cucumber: Cucumbers are loaded with gel water in and of themselves. We use them especially in the first two days of the program.

Ghee: Ghee is a clarified butter, heated until dairy particles are boiled off. This leaves behind butyric acid, an important fatty acid that plays a role in gut health. But there is more: Tests conducted by the Pollack Lab show that ghee has as high a concentration of gel water as chia seeds.

Ginger root: Ginger supports fast and effective kidney filtering and activates faster insulin uptake, sparing your cells from extra work.

Honey, raw: Honey is both a humectant and a demulcent, meaning it is a natural hydrator increasing moisture. A humectant seals in moisture, and a demulcent brings in moisture.

Lemons: Both lemons and limes contain pectin. Pectin is famous for making jams gel. Both are abundant in natural electrolytes. They replenish your body's mineral supply and quench your thirst more readily than plain water, precisely because the mineral agents regulate how water is transferred into the cell. The calcium, potassium, and magnesium are the key minerals acting as regulators of the electrical impulses that keep our body running.

Limes: Limes contains high amounts of hydrogen, which aids the body in gel formation through mineral charge, edging out lemon by just a bit.

Maple syrup: Maple syrup is full of minerals and a surprising amount of antioxidants, comparable even to a serving of berries.

Pears: Pears are a surprising source of fiber; there are almost six grams in a medium-sized pear. This combination of absorbing fiber and juiciness holds hydration and keeps water from flash-flooding our system.

Pomegranate juice: Pomegranates have 82 percent water content perfectly paired with potassium, a nutrient needed to pull hydration in past the cell wall. A half cup of pomegranate juice has more than 14 percent of the daily requirement of vitamin C.

Raspberries: Raspberries have eight grams of fiber per cup and are full of pectin. They are a member of the rose family; roses are also known for their high pectin content.

Salt: Sea salts and rock salts, unlike processed table salt, helps pull hydration into cells by providing necessary trace minerals without swelling and bloating.

Tea: We use chamomile and/or licorice tea, which may help with sleep and bloating.

Water!: Spring water or mineral waters come with minerals naturally embedded in them. Filtered and distilled water lack them. Simply add a pinch of sea salt or rock salt to a serving of filtered or distilled water.

Sweeten the Deal

You go for a sweetener these days at your local restaurant, and you are bombarded with choices: regular white table sugar (sucrose); artificial sweeteners like aspartame (Equal), sucralose (Splenda), and saccharin (Sweet & Low); and if you are at a more upscale or organic place, natural sugars like stevia, agave, raw sugar, and honey are also in the mix. What to choose?

Well, it is best to steer clear of all of them, but some of us need a little sweetness in our lives. So if you are going for it, go for the good stuff. Natural or raw is the way to go, and with good reason. Natural sugars, which usually come from fruit, hold on to healthy minerals and fiber. As with any sugar, consumption should be limited and in moderation. We realize some of these ingredients may be difficult to find, but they are increasingly more popular as a natural choice, so we decided to include them.

What should you avoid? We do not recommend artificial sweeteners. PERIOD. Nor are we fans of agave—even though it's lower on the glycemic index, it actually has more calories than sugar and may contain more than 70 percent fructose, which is more than what is in high-fructose corn syrup. Plus, its effects haven't been adequately studied yet. Just steer clear.

What should you use?

Stevia: Stevia, extracted from leaves of the stevia plant, is, in our opinion, the best choice of sweetener for anyone, even those with blood sugar problems. It has zero calories and no effect on blood sugar. However, there is a bitter aftertaste, so we suggest starting with tiny amounts and working up slowly to desired tastes. Many find liquid stevia more to their liking.

Raw organic honey: While honey is higher in fructose, it also has a good amount of antioxidants and is completely unprocessed, so it still retains all its nutritional value, unlike most store-bought honey. It's also been reported that honey may alleviate allergy symptoms!

Maple syrup: This is high (although not as high as table sugar) on the glycemic index, but it's loaded with antioxidants and minerals. Use in moderation. And make sure it's pure from real maple trees—the darker the color, the bolder the flavor. It is graded by the intensity of color and flavor, not by its mineral content, so choose what your taste buds prefer.

Blackstrap molasses: This thick and dark liquid is made from refined sugarcane. It's rich in iron and minerals, especially calcium and magnesium, and is lower on the glycemic index than sugar. It's a bit of an acquired taste.

Panela/raspadura/piloncillo: A traditional sugar popular in Latin countries, panela (or its alternative names) is unrefined cane sugar made from dehydrating sugarcane, so the minerals and antioxidants remain. It still has the same number of calories as table sugar, but it's better for you because of the intact nutrients. But do use sparingly.

Jaggery: Popular in India and other Asian countries, jaggery comes from the sap of palm trees as well as sugarcane (similar to panella). Sweet and unrefined, it's rich in minerals like iron.

Maguey sap: Hailing from Mexico, this fiber-rich sugar is a little hard to find, but it will sure impress your friends. It's an unrefined sweetener made from the agave plant, so it contains a lot of antioxidants and has a lot of prebiotic fiber, which provides nourishment to our healthy gut bacteria.

Licorice: Did you know that licorice is about fifty times as sweet as sugar and is zero on the glycemic index? It tastes like…well, licorice, but it's acceptable for diabetics, so that is a big plus. This may not seem like a ringing endorsement, but licorice is a good option as a sweetener; it just has a distinctive taste.

Monk fruit, or lo han guo: This is a fruit found in Southeast Asia. Its extract has gained popularity as a sugar substitute in the last few years, as it has zero calories and is 150 times sweeter than sugar (yes, we typed that right). It's high in antioxidants and low on the glycemic index—and tastes great.

Note: If you are diabetic or have blood sugar problems, you should consult with your doctor or nutritionist on which sugars are best for you.

MEAL IDEAS

Along with our hydration plan, we provide simple ideas and suggestions for good, healthy eating habits that you may want to follow during the five-day plan. With this hydration program, you can be vegan or paleo as your preferences prescribe, you can eat what you like and stop when you're full, but you will amplify the plan's health benefits by following the simple guidelines below that match your preferred diet.

Do eat:

- Fruits—a good rule of thumb with fruits is to stick to the lower glycemic fruits like berries, peaches, plums, grapefruit, kiwi, and melon. More exotic fruits like papaya, mango, pineapple, and banana have higher sugar content, so choose them less often. Skip using a banana in your smoothies, or go to half a one if you can't manage without. Better yet, substitute half an avocado, which has even more potassium than a banana. Or go deep and substitute a half cup of mashed sweet potato, a surprisingly tasty replacement.
- Greens and cooked and raw veggies
- Soups, which, of course, are another hydrating strategy. See our recipe section for some good choices, and stay away from store-bought canned and boxed soups—they have *way* too much sodium.
- Nuts and legumes. Mix up your nuts for variety. Soaking your beans before you cook them helps get rid of lectins, which can be harmful.
- Fish, best if wild caught

Will eating organic lead to better hydration?

Yes! Eating organic has a big advantage over conventionally raised fruits and veggies for hydration. You are not bringing in the pesticides typically sprayed on conventional crops, so your hydration doesn't have to be used to try to flush out so many chemicals. Most organics are raised with more nutrients in the soils, especially minerals. Those minerals are key to helping hydration become absorbed by the body. In addition, minerals collaborate with the water molecule to create energy for the body. Yet so many key minerals are missing from monocropped soils. When farmers pay attention, as organic farmers must, to soil health, minerals become available to us again through our foods. The benefit to us is not only more nutrition but more efficient and energizing hydration. If you can't eat organic, consider taking a trace mineral supplement. You can also check out the Resources section for the Environmental Working Group's list of which fruits and veggies should not be eaten if not organic and which ones you can be a little lenient about when buying.

Some foods require more hydration in order to be fully digested, so we recommend you avoid the following list:

- Simple carbohydrates like pasta and bread
- Processed foods
- Added sugar
- Trans fats
- Hydrogenated and partially hydrogenated oils
- Fake sweeteners like sucralose, saccharine, and aspartame

Fish
Some fish, like marlin, tuna, shark, swordfish, and mackerel, have higher concentrations of mercury than others, so be careful when selecting your fish, especially if you are pregnant or have children. See NRDC.org for the Natural Resource Defense Council's Smart Seafood Buying Guide for mercury content in fish.

Last but certainly not least, liquid water should still be part of your diet. If you need to, sip water throughout the day to quench your thirst. You don't need to salt every time you drink. Also, as part of the Quench Plan, drink a cup or two of water before every meal.

MEALS

The following are great suggestions for meals throughout the day so that you can bring even more hydrating foods into your routine. Also, once you are done with the five-day plan, see our recipes in the next chapter, "The Cup Runneth Over," for some great recipes.

Breakfast Suggestions

You may find the smoothie is sufficient for some meals, but if you are still hungry, here are some good ideas for breakfast.

- Eggs any style—try over sautéed greens like spinach, kale, or collards

- Steel-cut oatmeal / cream of rice / hot millet with almond slivers and cranberries
- Smoked salmon with capers and pickled onions
- Piece of fruit slathered with nut butter
- Leftovers are a great idea for breakfast. Who said breakfast can't be savory? We often purposely leave some of our dinner plate over to wrap up for breakfast the next day. Salmon with beurre blanc is actually delicious cold and kills two birds with one stone—fewer calories for dinner, and breakfast is already prepared!

Lunch Suggestions

- Grilled chicken or salmon over salad
- Bean salad in radicchio or romaine "cups"
- Sautéed escarole—add canned cannellini beans, drizzle with extra-virgin olive oil, and sprinkle with parmigiana cheese
- Niçoise salad—hard-boiled egg, flaked tuna, green beans, radish over greens
- Chicken, veggie, and/or bean/lentil soup

Dinner Suggestions

Have one of each category:

- Protein of your choice: beef—preferably grass-fed—organic chicken, turkey, pork, wild-caught fish (try to have at least twice a week), beans
- Small side salad, even if just iceberg lettuce with olive oil and pinch of salt, oregano, and a dash of red wine vinegar. Add any other veggies you like, of course.

- Side of veggies: A simple favorite of Dana's is broccoli sautéed in macadamia nut oil (delicious and buttery) with a pinch of sea salt.
- Can have ½ cup of unprocessed starch side, like brown rice, quinoa, or yam

Snack Suggestions

- Hummus and celery, carrots, and/or bell peppers
- Handful of nuts—any will do—or spoonful of a nut butter
- Bone broth, a favorite of ours. You can sip it throughout the day if you have a heat-retaining thermos. (See recipe in chapter 9.)
- One half avocado with squeeze of a lime wedge and pinch of sea salt
- Olives; about ten is a good snack size

FIVE-DAY QUENCH PLAN

Day One

Remember to have 1 to 2 cups of water before every meal. Of course if you are drinking a smoothie as a meal replacement, it isn't necessary. Try room temperature or even hot water to see if you prefer it.

Morning Micromovement

When you wake, reclose your eyes. Don't join the world yet; savor the transition. Register how you feel and see if you notice a difference five days from now. Relish the coming changes.

Do our Chin Meets Chest exercise, which uses your average ten-pound head as a priming weight to pump fluids throughout your spinal canal. You've now squeezed out toxins released from your brain during your sleep and replaced them with fresh nutrients and oxygen. Not to mention your abs get worked, all while lying down.

Chin Meets Chest: Arrange yourself flat on your back, your head on your pillow, and become aware of your spine from bottom to top. If you find the position uncomfortable, try it on your side. Simply lower your chin toward your chest, stretching comfortably. Feel the gentle pull up the back of your neck. Hold it for two deep breaths. Do not strain: You are moving fluids, not exerting muscles. After two breaths, slowly raise your chin back up, keeping your neck muscles relaxed. Repeat this movement three times. Do more it you like, but don't overdo it. Studies show we quit easily if we push too hard in the beginning. Chin Meets Chest is a great move to use when you are standing.

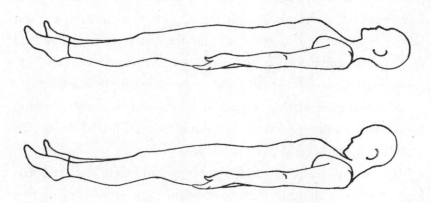

Morning Beverage

Upon rising, drink 8 to 16 ounces of warm or tepid water with juice from a lemon wedge. You can also use a teaspoon or two of apple cider vinegar (the cap from the bottle measures out a teaspoon exactly) or add some crushed fresh or dried mint leaves, a sprig of rosemary, or a chamomile tea bag. These additions release essential oils and substances that help your body absorb the water. Again, our program is not about drinking as much as possible but maximizing hydration. Drink the amount that feels comfortable to you, an amount that will keep you returning to the practice, not avoiding it.

If you regularly have coffee or tea first thing in the morning, please limit yourself to 1 or 2 cups. Don't use coffee only to hydrate. Just make sure to get that glass of lemon water into you early in the morning. Still, a trick for making your coffee more hydrating is to blend a teaspoon of unsalted grass-fed butter and/or a teaspoon of coconut oil into your hot beverage. This is a very ancient endurance drink, based on classic Himalayan, Ethiopian, and Peruvian techniques. Bulletproof coffee, a modern version of this, has become widely popular for good reason. Blending makes this coffee a truly wonderful latte. The added oils help move hydration into the cells and can even buffer caffeine jitters.

Morning Smoothie: Choose either a cold-weather smoothie for winter months, such as Warming Sweet Nut Milk, or the warm-weather version of Lime-Aid.

If you want to be super efficient, you can batch your smoothies by prepping all your ingredients at the same time. Line up five heavy ziplock plastic bags or, even better, glass jars or containers, and add all the ingredients for one smoothie per container, except the liquids, and refrigerate. Then freshly blend one each morning with the required liquid. It's best to blend daily for the freshest taste and nutrients, but you can also prepare your smoothie the night before, which will result in a modest reduction in nutrition.

Drink your smoothie within two hours of waking. You could drink it on your way to work or take it on a morning walk, or just drink it while reading the morning news.

Warm-Weather Smoothies: Lime-Aid

The ingredients in this recipe synergize to create more efficient hydration. Chia has the ability to release the most water of any nutritious seed.

MAKES APPROXIMATELY A 12-OUNCE SERVING

½ cup coconut water or coconut milk (no sugar added)
½ cucumber, peeled, if not organic
1 tablespoon ground chia seeds
1 to 2 teaspoons honey
1 tablespoon fresh lime juice
1 to 2 pinches coarse sea salt or rock salt (such as Himalayan pink salt)
1 to 2 cups spring or filtered water, dilute to your taste preference
½ to 1 teaspoon minced fresh ginger, optional if you want
    extra zip

Place ingredients in blender and blend on high. Pour over ice if desired.

Cool-Weather Option: Warming Sweet Nut Milk

The nuts add fat, fiber, and protein, and the ginger and cardamom add a bright flavor.

MAKES APPROXIMATELY A 12-OUNCE SERVING

1 tablespoon ground chia seeds

½ cup coconut milk (no sugar added)

2 tablespoons ground cashews or any ground nut or seed such as
hemp, sunflower, or pumpkin

1 to 2 teaspoons maple syrup or stevia (to taste)

1 teaspoon fresh diced ginger

¼ teaspoon ground cardamom or ground cinnamon

1 to 2 pinches unrefined sea or rock salt (such as Himalayan
pink salt)

1 cup filtered or spring water, or more to dilute to your taste

If you can't find ground chia seeds or don't want to grind your own (we use a coffee grinder), you can toss them whole in your blender. They will still release their gel. They may be a crunchy texture before they get fully saturated. If you don't like the crunch, you can soak seeds 5 minutes in advance, while you prepare the rest of the smoothie. To soak, use 3 tablespoons of water to 1 tablespoon of chia seeds, add it all back into smoothie.

Place in blender and blend. Pour into a cup or thermos. Some people are tempted to add their coffee to their smoothie. Go ahead.

Do follow the blender manufacturer's instructions on hot water in blenders. Some may caution you not blend hot liquids but add to other ingredients after blending.

Midday Movement

Spinal Twists: Sit on the edge of a chair at your office or home. Hold your arms straight out to the sides with your palms facing up, and gently rotate your whole upper body to the right. Keep your hips planted forward, and turn your torso, arms, and head in unison. Let your eyes follow your thumb. Rotate your thumbs back and forth. Repeat to the left. Do three full twists.

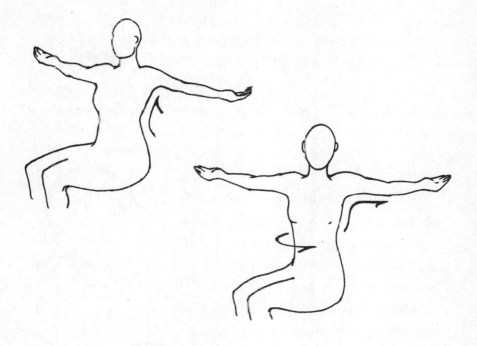

Afternoon Delight

Fill a sixteen-ounce bottle with fourteen ounces of spring or filtered water and a pinch of sea salt. Add two tablespoons of ground chia seed and shake vigorously. Add two tablespoons of an unsweetened fruit juice or juice concentrates, such as pomegranate, concord grape, cherry, or blueberry. Either juice or the harder-to-find concentrates work well; it's your preference. What is great about concentrates is they can last longer without refrigeration, so you can keep them in your desk or car. Health food stores are more likely to carry concentrates. You don't have to consume your Afternoon Delight all at once. Simply finish it by the end of the workday. Drink at your pace between noon and seven p.m.

Bedtime Beverage

Chamomile tea has long been used to promote relaxation, and it also helps detoxification during sleep. Licorice tea is a good alternative to chamomile; its sweetness makes it an end of day reward. We recommend just a half cup, four ounces, at nighttime.

Bedtime Movement

Ear Meets Shoulder: Sit on the edge of your bed. Gently roll your neck from your right ear to your right shoulder, and then repeat on the left side. Start with five on each side.

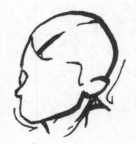

Chin Circles: Then use your chin and draw a circle in the air. Do five circles.

Full Body Stretch: Lie down and stretch your whole body in a gentle elongating movement, for the count of five breaths. Then raise your arms overhead and bend them a little behind you so that you can grip the headboard or mattress

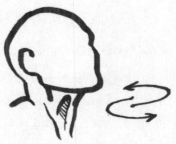

edge, and pull to elongate your torso and abdomen between hips and ribs, release, and relax. Try two, three, or five times. Good night, sleep well.

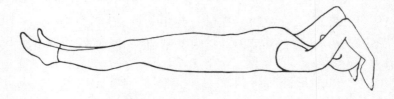

Day Two

Morning Micromovement

Practice your awakening routine as in Day One: After you awaken, reclose your eyes and notice your spine. Feel its warm length after a night's sleep. Do Chin Meets Chest for two deep breaths; repeat three times. Now do Shoulders Massage Bed.

Shoulders Massage Bed: Lie on your back and gently press your right shoulder blade into the mattress. You can experiment by lifting either elbow to help. Press for two deep breaths and release. Repeat with the left shoulder blade for two deep breaths. You may notice one side is easier to do than the other, and that lets you know where you might want to help your body strengthen by doing a few more moves on the weaker side. There is no perfect execution of our moves because fluid is so, well, fluid. Just enjoy finding new moves; no matter what, you are getting hydration delivered to new places.

Morning Beverages

Upon rising, drink 8 to 16 ounces of warm or tepid water with juice from a lemon wedge. You can also use apple cider vinegar instead of lemon, or add a few leaves of mint or a sprig of rosemary, or a tea bag of chamomile. If your morning must include coffee or tea, please limit your intake to 1 or 2 cups, and consider blending in a teaspoon of grass-fed butter or coconut oil or a little of both to make your coffee a hydrating drink.

Morning Smoothie: Choose the hot or cold recipe, and today add ½ cup fresh or frozen raspberries for a fresh, new taste. Raspberries are loaded with antioxidants and also give fiber for better absorption of fluid into your tissues.

Midday Movement

Thumb Presses Sternum: You can do this sitting or standing. Breathe through your nose, mouth closed, and place one hand flat on your upper torso, with your thumb on your sternum, right between your nipples. Inhale slowly to the count of five; then press your hand in as if pushing air out of a ziplock bag as you exhale through your 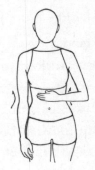 nose. Do it gently and slowly to the count of five. Repeat three times. This exercise both reminds you to breathe and pumps fluids further to your organs.

The diaphragm, right under your sternum, is the main muscle of respiration, and it pulls in a significant amount of hydrating vapor from the air. A deep exhale massages and stimulates both the liver and the stomach and increases lung capacity. Now do your Spinal Twists.

Afternoon Delight

Repeat the recipe from Day One. If you want a little variety, use 2 ounces of a different unsweetened juice or concentrate.

Bedtime Beverage

Chamomile or licorice tea (½ cup)

Bedtime Movement

Ear Meets Shoulder, Chin Circles, and Full Body Stretch

Day Three

Morning Movement

After you awaken, reclose your eyes and notice your spine. Then practice your awakening routine of Chin Meets Chest and Shoulders Massage Bed.

Next we add a great new stretch called a Cat Back.

Cat Back: Sit on the edge of your bed with your feet on the floor, knees apart in a V shape, just so you're comfortable. Place your hands on your knees. Sit tall, gently lean over—do not exceed your comfort level. Inhale as you let your chin float out past your knees and then look at the floor. Bring your shoulders near your ears and draw your chin into your chest. Exhale as you straighten your arms and roll yourself back into sitting straight. Bonus: Curve your back into a C shape and rock back and forth. Repeat twice.

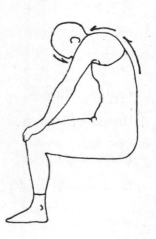

Morning Beverages

Drink 8 to 16 ounces of warm or tepid water with juice from a lemon quarter. You can also add fresh mint leaves, a sprig of rosemary, or a chamomile tea bag. If you are drinking morning coffee, consider blending a pat of grass-fed butter and a teaspoon of coconut oil. It whips into a wonderful latte, and you've just made your coffee a powerhouse hydrator. Adding butter or coconut oil or milk to tea works too. Indeed this is typical practice in high-altitude environments around the world and is considered an endurance drink. Top with cinnamon or cardamom.

Morning Smoothie: Choose the hot or cold recipe, and for variety today add half a pear. Pears are a great source of fiber and a top hydrating fruit.

Midday Movement

Thumb Presses Sternum and Spinal Twists

Afternoon Delight

Follow the instructions for the recipe from Day One with any variety of juice you prefer.

Bedtime Beverage

Chamomile or licorice tea (½ cup)

Bedtime Movement

Ear Meets Shoulder, Chin Circles, and Full Body Stretch

Day Four

Morning Movement

Practice your awakening routine with Chin Meets Chest, Shoulders Massage Bed, and Cat Back.

Morning Beverages

Drink 8 to 16 ounces of warm or tepid water with the juice from a lemon quarter. You can also add fresh mint leaves, a sprig of rosemary, or a chamomile tea bag. If you are drinking morning coffee, consider blending a pat of grass-fed butter and a teaspoon of coconut oil. Top with cinnamon or cardamom.

Morning Smoothie: Choose the hot or cold recipe, but for variety today blend in 2 tablespoons of alfalfa sprouts. Though tasteless, and you will never notice, sprouts bring a bang of gel, vitamins, and minerals to the mix. It's a great way to sneak greens into unsuspecting mouths.

Midday Movement

Thumb Presses Sternum and Spinal Twists

Afternoon Delight

Follow the instructions for Day One, and add unsweetened juice or concentrate as you like.

Bedtime Beverage

Chamomile or licorice tea (½ cup)

Bedtime Movement

Ear Meets Shoulders, Chin Circles, and Full Body Stretch

Day Five

Morning Movement

Practice your awakening routine with Chin Meets Chest and Shoulders Massage Bed.

We're going to do a variation of the Cat Back today. This move is called Snake Out in the dance world.

Snake Out: Sit on the edge of your bed with your feet on the floor, knees apart slightly in a V shape so you're comfortable. Place your hands on your knees. Sit tall, and with a straight back lean over until your head is between your knees or as far as feels gentle and comfortable for you. This time, when you start to rise by straightening your arms, as in Cat Back, instead raise your head up slowly so that, as you are sitting back up, you look forward first at the wall in front of you and then up at the ceiling. Then gently arch your back. Allow your eyes to slowly move all the way up the wall toward the ceiling and stretch your neck back in a con- trolled movement. You may want to support your back as you rise by pressing your hands on your knees to help you return to a sitting posi- tion, then release. Practice a nice rolling movement. Repeat for three rounds.

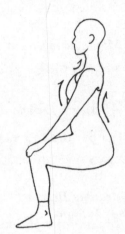

Morning Beverages

Drink 8 to 16 ounces of warm or tepid water with juice from a lemon wedge. You can also add mint, rosemary, or even a tea bag of chamomile. If your morn- ing must include coffee or tea, 1 or 2 cups is fine; consider add- ing a teaspoon of grass-fed butter or coconut oil.

Morning Smoothie: Choose the hot or cold recipe, and for variety today add 2 tablespoons of one of the concentrates or fruit juices from the Afternoon Delight recipe (see Why Our Shopping List Is So Hydrating in chapter 8).

Midday Movement

Thumb Presses Sternum and Spinal Twists

Afternoon Delight

Repeat the recipe from Day One with a juice or concentrate of your choice.

Bedtime Beverage

Chamomile or licorice tea (½ cup)

Bedtime Movement

Ear Meets Shoulder, Chin Circles, and Full Body Stretch

Congratulations! You have completed the five-day program. You now know what it feels like to be optimally hydrated and keep your own self fluid through the day in our modern dehydrating world. If you continue the principles of Quench, in one month you will have accelerated your waste removal on all fronts, which will continue to improve your skin, brain, joints, and muscles. If you keep going for three months, you will likely experience easier weight loss as well as clearer thinking, enhanced mood, improved agility and range of motion, and deeper sleep. You will be feeling it: your new younger self.

5-DAY QUENCH PROGRAM AT-A-GLANCE

	Day 1	Day 2	Day 3	Day 4	Day 5
Morning Micro-movement	Chin Meets Chest	Chin Meets Chest, Shoulders Massage Bed	Chin Meets Chest, Shoulders Massage Bed, and Cat Back	Chin Meets Chest, Shoulders Massage Bed, and Cat Back	Chin Meets Chest, Shoulders Massage Bed, and Snake Out

	Day 1	*Day 2*	*Day 3*	*Day 4*	*Day 5*
Morning Beverage	Warm water with lemon	Warm water with lemon	Warm water with lemon	Warm water with lemon	Warm water with lemon
Morning Smoothie	Lime-Aid or Warming Sweet Nut Milk	Lime-Aid or Warming Sweet Nut Milk, with raspberries	Lime-Aid or Warming Sweet Nut Milk, with pear	Lime-Aid or Warming Sweet Nut Milk, with sprouts	Lime-Aid or Warming Sweet Nut Milk, with pomegranate (or other) juice
Midday Micro-movement	Spinal Twists	Thumb Presses Sternum and Spinal Twists	Thumb Presses Sternum and Spinal Twists	Thumb Presses Sternum and Spinal Twists	Thumb Presses Sternum and Spinal Twists
Afternoon Beverage	Afternoon Delight	Afternoon Delight	Afternoon Delight	Afternoon Delight	Afternoon Delight
Bedtime Beverage	Chamomile or licorice tea	Chamomile or licorice tea	Chamomile or licorice tea	Chamomile or licorice tea	Chamomile or licorice tea
Bedtime Micro-movement	Ear Meets Shoulder, Chin Circles, and Full Body Stretch	Ear Meets Shoulder, Chin Circles, and Full Body Stretch	Ear Meets Shoulder, Chin Circles, and Full Body Stretch	Ear Meets Shoulder, Chin Circles, and Full Body Stretch	Ear Meets Shoulder, Chin Circles, and Full Body Stretch

CHAPTER 9

The Cup Runneth Over

Recipes for a Lifetime

Eat deliberately, with other people whenever possible, and always with pleasure.

—*Michael Pollan*

So you've experienced the five-day plan—do you feel buoyant? More energetic? Less aches and pains? No more headaches? Less bloating? Want to make it your life? Great! In this section you get more delicious and healthy smoothie recipes and as well as other great suggestions for soups, light meals, and desserts (including popsicles!) that will help you stay running smooth at optimal hydration.

With that in mind, we made another handy chart for you that incorporates our meal recipes with drinks, smoothies, and micromovements to follow. Please feel free to mix and match with any of the recipes. We hope you notice you are naturally practicing micromovements throughout your day because it feels great and that you now seek drinking as a matter of course.

BEYOND 5: A TYPICAL WEEK ON THE PROGRAM

	Day 1	Day 2	Day 3	Day 4	Day 5
Morning Micro-movement	Chin Meets Chest	Chin Meets Chest and Shoulders Massage Bed	Chin Meets Chest and Shoulders Massage Bed	Chin Meets Chest, Shoulders Massage Bed, and Cat Back	Chin Meets Chest, Shoulders Massage Bed, and Snake Out
Morning Beverage	Warm water with lemon	Warm water with lemon	Warm water with lemon	Warm water with lemon	Warm water with lemon
Morning Smoothie	Lime-Aid or Warming Sweet Nut Milk	Pineapple-Ginger Smoothie	Blueberry-Avocado Smoothie	Lime-Aid or Warming Sweet Nut Milk	Green Detox Smoothie
Breakfast	Avocado nest	Bowl of fruit	Salmon with capers	Steel-cut oatmeal	Chia pudding
Lunch	Chicken over arugula	Soup of your choice	Three-bean salad	Soup of your choice	Zucchini spiral noodles
Midday Micro-movement	Spinal Twists	Thumb Presses Sternum and Spinal Twists	Thumb Presses Sternum and Spinal Twists	Thumb Presses Sternum and Spinal Twists	Thumb Presses Sternum and Spinal Twists
Snack	Nuts	Cup of bone broth	Cup of olives	Hummus with veggies	½ avocado
Afternoon Beverage	Afternoon Delight	Afternoon Delight	Afternoon Delight	Afternoon Delight	Afternoon Delight
Dinner	Cauliflower steak	Broiled fish with quinoa	Roasted chicken with veggies	Niçoise salad	Mushroom arugula mash
Bedtime Beverage	Chamomile or licorice tea	Chamomile or licorice tea	Chamomile or licorice tea	Chamomile or licorice tea	Chamomile or licorice tea

	Day 1	Day 2	Day 3	Day 4	Day 5
Bedtime Micro-movement	Ear Meets Shoulder, Chin Circles, and Full Body Stretch	Ear Meets Shoulder, Chin Circles, and Full Body Stretch	Ear Meets Shoulder, Chin Circles, and Full Body Stretch	Ear Meets Shoulder, Chin Circles, and Full Body Stretch	Ear Meets Shoulder, Chin Circles, and Full Body Stretch

Smoothies, the heart of the Quench Plan—what else can we say—are the most perfect hydrating drinks. So we give you plenty of options here. Each smoothie has just the right amount of absorptive nutrition to keep you going ... and going ... and going! Experiment—use other berries, greens, and good fruits to make these your own. And invest in a good travel container so you are never without.

By the way, there are easy tricks for making smoothies even more nourishing—make them into fermented drinks. Add raw apple cider vinegar, hot sauces, miso paste, or just break open a probiotic capsule. All these, when ingested with adequate hydration, help the bacteria function quickly and optimally.

BLENDERS 101

A lion's share of the recipes in the Quench Plan are made with blenders. These days there are many great brands and models on the market—so many that it may be hard to choose from. From down-and-dirty, one-serving machines to pricey deluxe restaurant-grade contraptions, we have tested them all. First think about your budget, the size of your kitchen, and your gadget skills. While the high-speed, high-priced blenders will smooth your smoothie to perfection, we emphasize that any blender will get you started with our hydration plan, and we just want to get you feeling better. If your cheapo blender gives you a gritty smoothie, you can pass it through a strainer to get it to a more palatable state. Even if you lose some of that important fiber, you are still boosting your hydration factor.

Our suggestions: For simplicity and ease, we like Nutri-Bullet, since it blends in a portable container. Zip and go. In addition, it grinds seeds and nuts beautifully, but it especially grinds chia seeds nice and fine, getting the most gel release out of the powder. Blendtec and Vitamix are high-speed blenders with great reputations, but they may be out of your budget.

A special note on old-fashioned Osterizers. This is how we got our start. One unique advantage to Osterizers is that you can replace the glass pitcher with a special plastic Ball jar for single serving preparation that you can just cap and go. Osterizers were designed in the 1920s to speed labor-intensive canning, so upgrade that capacity to one-container cleanup. Or imagine five Ball jars lined up in your fridge, each with daily ingredients just waiting to be blended with liquid, hot or cold, and carried out the door. Super easy, not to mention beautiful.

Note: Allow any hot beverage (including coffee) to cool for a bit so the steam doesn't build up, causing the lid to pop off and scald you. Also, depending on the size of your blender, don't overfill. We've experienced overfill, and it isn't pretty. Blend in two sessions if you have to.

TIPS FOR MAKING SMOOTHIES
AND OTHER DRINKS

All of our recipes have been carefully created to provide you optimal hydration. We've paired ingredients to maximize the effects not only for nutrition but also for hydrating absorption.

- To create your own concoction that is extra hydrating, make sure it includes one or more leafy greens and/or herbs (98 percent gel water); a bit of fruit for sweetness; a healthy fat, like avocado, olive, or other good oils, or nuts and seeds; an acidic zing from lime juice or raw apple cider vinegar; and a final pinch of coarse sea salt.

- All the drink recipes make one serving unless otherwise noted but one man's serving is another man's overkill. Drink to *your* fill.

- When a recipe calls for chia seeds, buy ground or grind you own. Grinding makes them gel instantly when liquid is added. No need to presoak.

- It's okay to use frozen fruit (preferably organic) in these recipes. In fact, it makes it easier to always have fruit on hand. And frozen berries can be great if you make your smoothies at work, since they will last a whole week in a fridge.

- When making smoothies and other drinks, use filtered or spring water, mineral or sparkling. If you choose distilled, add salt or liquid minerals. (See the Resources section for the best filters for your budget.)

HOT-WEATHER BEVERAGES

The Foundation

Use this recipe as a guide for making cooling summer smoothies. For variety, try romaine lettuce in place of or in combination with spinach. Parsley, mint, basil, and celery are refreshing additions, too. For a hint of sweetness, why not toss in a pear or pumpkin puree instead of the apple? A pinch of fragrant cardamom gives another layer of flavor.

> 1 cup packed spinach
> ½ cucumber, peeled, if not organic
> 1 green apple, peeled, cored, and quartered
> Juice of ½ lime
> ½ cup coconut milk
> 1 to 2 teaspoons minced ginger
> 1 to 2 cups filtered or spring water, diluted to taste

Place all the ingredients in a blender, and secure the lid. Blend. Serve immediately.

Watermelon-Cucumber Splash

Watermelon and cucumber, which are botanical cousins, are on our list of top ten hydrating fruits and vegetables. Adding a pinch of salt enhances the electric charge. Using herbal teas, such as hibiscus or peppermint, in place of water adds to the flavor.

1 cup cubed watermelon

1 medium cucumber, peeled, if not organic

Squeeze of fresh lime juice

Pinch of coarse sea salt

1 or 2 cups filtered water or hibiscus tea, diluted to your
    preference

Mint sprig, optional

Place all the ingredients in a blender and secure the lid. Blend for 30 to 35 seconds or until desired consistency is reached. Serve immediately.

The Quench

You will need a high-powered blender for this drink, because fennel is hard to break down. But as one of our go-to smoothies, it is quenching, filling, and beautiful to look at. And this is one of many recipes in which we blend in chia seeds, a favorite Quench ingredient.

3 celery ribs

½ cucumber, peeled, if not organic

1 cup kale, spinach, or spring mix greens

½ fennel bulb

½ pear or apple, peeled, cored, and cut up

Juice of 1 lime

1 teaspoon to 1 tablespoon coconut oil or extra-virgin olive oil

½- to 1-inch piece ginger, depending on taste, diced

1 teaspoon to 1 tablespoon ground chia seeds

1 to 2 cups filtered, spring, or sparkling water, diluted to your
    preference

Place all the ingredients in a blender and secure the lid. Blend for 30 to 35 seconds or until desired consistency is reached. Serve immediately.

Berry Red Smoothie

You may think that red cabbage would overpower the other flavors in this smoothie, but it doesn't. It actually enhances the flavor of the raspberries.

  1 cup shredded red cabbage
  1 cup fresh or frozen raspberries
  ½ cucumber, peeled if not organic
  6 to 8 basil or mint leaves
  ½- to 1-inch piece ginger, depending on taste, diced
  1 teaspoon to 1 tablespoon coconut oil
  1 to 2 cups filtered, spring, or sparkling water, diluted to your
     preference
Freshly ground black pepper

Place all the ingredients, except the black pepper, in a blender and secure the lid. Blend for 30 to 35 seconds or until desired consistency is reached. Grind some pepper on top and serve immediately.

We Got the Beet

Beets have been used for their medicinal and nutritional benefits for thousands of years. Taken from the root of the flowering beet plant, beet powder is deep red and packed with nutrients and antioxidants. Be sure to purchase beet powder that has no added sugar. How much ginger you use is entirely up to you.

1 teaspoon to 1 tablespoon chia seeds (ground are best)

½ cup raw or cooked diced beet, or 1 tablespoon beet powder

1 cup (about 10) red grapes

1 cup watercress or arugula

¼ cup parsley, leaves and stems

1 teaspoon to 1 tablespoon coconut oil

½- to 1-inch piece ginger, diced

Pinch of coarse sea salt

1 to 2 cups filtered, spring, or sparkling water, diluted to your
  preference

Place ingredients in a blender and secure the lid. Blend for 30 to 35 seconds or until desired consistency is reached. Serve immediately.

Mango Colada

Mangos, while they are a high-glycemic food, benefit here from a hit of apple cider vinegar, which helps bring down the sugar impact.

1 teaspoon to 1 tablespoon chia seed (ground is best)

1 cup leafy greens, such as spinach, spring mix, romaine, or other
  lettuces

½ mango, peeled and cut up

½ cucumber, peeled if not organic

1 teaspoon raw apple cider vinegar

¼ cup cashews

1 teaspoon to 1 tablespoon coconut oil

6 to 8 basil leaves

1 to 2 cups filtered or spring water, adjusted for your preferred thickness

Place ingredients in a blender and secure the lid. Blend for 30 to 35 seconds or until desired consistency is reached. Serve immediately.

The Quench Detox

1 small raw or cooked beet, diced*

1 celery stalk

1 handful of parsley

1 cucumber, peeled if not organic

¼-inch piece ginger, diced

Juice of ½ lemon

4 romaine lettuce leaves

1 handful spinach or arugula

½ ripe pear

1 to 2 cups filtered or spring water, adjusted for your preferred
   thickness

Add all the ingredients and blend. Pour in a glass and enjoy.

If you use a raw beet, use a high-speed blender or dice very fine.

Pineapple-Mango Smoothie

1½ cups fresh or frozen pineapple cubes

1 cup fresh or frozen mango cubes

1 cup coconut water

1 celery rib, cut up

½-inch piece ginger, peeled

2 teaspoons raw apple cider vinegar

1 to 2 cups filtered or spring water, adjusted for your preferred
   thickness

Put all the ingredients into a blender and puree. Pour into a glass and
drink immediately.

Greenscape Detox Smoothie

1 tablespoon chia seeds
1 cup fresh or frozen pineapple cubes
¼ avocado
1 celery rib
½ cup basil leaves
½ cup parsley
½ cucumber, peeled, if not organic
1 to 2 teaspoons diced ginger
Juice of ½ lime
1 to 2 cups filtered or spring water, adjusted for your preferred
    thickness

Put all the ingredients into a blender and puree. Pour into a glass and drink immediately.

Blueberry-Avocado Smoothie

1½ cups fresh or frozen blueberries
½ avocado, peeled and pitted
1 apple or 1 pear, halved and cored
1 to 2 cups filtered or spring water, adjusted for your preferred
    thickness

Put all the ingredients into a blender and puree. Pour into a glass and drink immediately.

Golden Smoothie

2 apples, quartered and cored

3 oranges, peeled

Juice of ½ lemon

1 cup coconut water

½-inch piece fresh ginger, peeled

¼-inch piece fresh turmeric or ⅛ teaspoon ground

1 or 2 cups filtered or spring water, adjusted for your preferred
thickness

Put all the ingredients into a blender and puree. Pour into a glass and drink immediately.

Raspberry Smoothie

1 cup fresh or frozen raspberries

2 oranges, peeled

½ avocado

1 handful basil

½ cup coconut water

1 to 2 cups filtered or spring water, adjusted for your preferred
thickness

Put all the ingredients into a blender and puree. Pour into a glass and drink immediately.

COLD-WEATHER BEVERAGES

When the leaves start to change and you find yourself leaving the house with a sweater, it's time to switch to warming hot drinks. Though we more naturally think to hydrate in summer, winter months require just as much hydration. Our recipes often mix savory with sweet, an enticing taste combination that tempts us to drink more and results in better hydration and immune protection during this drying season.

Remember to fill the blender less than half full when blending hot liquids to prevent explosions. Follow each blender manufacturer's instructions on blending heated ingredients, as they are all different.

Bergamot Coconut Tea

Fragrant bergamot is a small greenish citrus fruit that imparts a distinctive scent to Earl Grey tea. It recently has been shown to be a powerful tool in lowering cholesterol in humans.[1]

1 cup brewed Earl Grey tea
¼ cup coconut milk
¼ cup ground raw cashews
Pinch of coarse sea salt

Blend for 30 to 35 seconds or until desired consistency is reached. Add more hot water if you prefer a thinner consistency. Consider sweetening with maple syrup. Serve immediately.

Basil Lemon Tea

While honey is a good humectant, stevia or lo han guo fruit (also called monk fruit) are good low-glycemic substitutes. Lo han guo can be found at a health food store in powdered form. Although basil tea is known all over the world, it is known as holy tea in India, called Tulsi. The tea's herbal properties are believed to reduce stress. If you don't have basil, use fresh mint; basil and lemon can also be added to licorice tea for a rich, satisfying flavor combination.

3 to 5 basil leaves

1 cup boiling water

1 teaspoon honey

1 teaspoon fresh lemon juice or to taste

Put the basil leaves in a cup. Add the water, then stir in the honey and lemon juice. Sip while hot.

Persian Rose Tea

Rose petals have been used to hold hydration since ancient times. Rose petal tea can be purchased at health food stores or online. We add a bit of miso, a fermented soybean paste, known for its probiotic (healthy gut bacteria) benefits and to further retain moisture. This recipe is a standout when you add a teaspoon of rose petal jam, which can be found in gourmet or Middle Eastern grocery stores. You can also sweeten with the maple syrup listed in the recipe. It is a good hydrating agent, or powdered or liquid stevia can be used in a small amount instead. (*Note:* If you have never used powdered stevia, start with a tiny amount—less than ⅛ teaspoon—to find your taste preference.) The cayenne adds anti-inflammatory properties and a hint of zingy flavor.

1 cup rose petal tea, steeped for 5 minutes

1 teaspoon red or white miso paste

1 teaspoon maple syrup

Pinch of cayenne pepper

Prepare the tea. Stir the miso, maple syrup, and cayenne into the hot tea. Sip while hot.

Wu Wei Cuppa Miso

Wu Wei tea, a great mix of Asian herbs and spices, can be bought at your local health food store. When mixed with miso, it makes a lovely savory and sweet taste. This recipe can also be made with rose petal tea. It is really outstanding when you add ½ teaspoon of rose petal jam.

    1 cup Wu Wei tea, steeped for 5 minutes
    ½ to 1 teaspoon white miso paste

Prepare the tea. Stir the miso into the hot tea to dissolve. Sip while hot.

Apple Cider–Orange Sour

Sounds like a fancy cocktail, doesn't it? This is based on an Early American recipe called shrug, used widely in the colonial days to fend off colds.

    1 cup hot water
    Juice of 1 orange
    ½ teaspoon raw apple cider vinegar
    ¼ teaspoon powdered ginger. You can use fresh grated ginger, but it
        will be gritty. Another trick can be to use a splash of the the new
        liquid ginger shots showing up all over health-conscious stores.

Put all the ingredients into a blender and blend for 5 to 10 seconds, following the blender manufacturer's directions for hot liquids. This drink can also be mixed without a blender. Sip while hot. This can also be a great drink in the summer, replacing the hot water with cold.

Coconut-Tahini with Espresso

Coconut milk and cocoa powder are a classic combination. Adding espresso and tahini take it to a new hydrating level.

6 ounces coconut milk

2 teaspoons unsweetened cocoa powder

2 ounces hot brewed espresso

1 ounce hot water

1½ tablespoons tahini

1 tablespoon maple syrup

Pinch of sea salt

Put all the ingredients into a blender and blend for 30 to 35 seconds, following the blender manufacturer's instructions for hot liquids. Enjoy while hot.

Coffee?

Everyone seems to want to know about the connection between coffee and hydration. Good news for coffee drinkers: The available studies on hydration found that caffeine intakes up to 400 milligrams per day (about 4 cups of brewed coffee) did not produce dehydration. However, just for the five-day Quench Plan, we recommend one coffee a day, because those other cups should be filled with more hydrating liquids. During the Quench Plan, for you guzzlers out there who drink four to six cups or more, this can have a diuretic effect and therefore deplete your body of hydration. So just take it easy with the double espressos. You probably already know if you are one of those bodies that can tolerate coffee or not.

All that said, here is the biggest new study on coffee, showing it lowers all-cause mortality: M. J. Gunter et al., "Coffee Drinking and Mortality in 10 European Countries: A Multinational Cohort Study," *Annuals of Internal Medicine* 167, no. 4 (August 2017): 236–247.

Reishi Coffee

Reishi mushrooms have been used in the Americas, Japan, Vietnam, and China for many medicinal purposes, including immune system enhancement and better sleep. The powder can be purchased online and in health food stores. If you wish. add some ground cardamom or cinnamon or a bit of vanilla.

    1 cup hot strong coffee
    ¼ to ½ teaspoon powdered reishi mushroom
    1 teaspoon butter
    2 teaspoons maple syrup

Blend half the cup of coffee with mushroom, butter, and syrup. Pour into a cup and add the rest of the coffee. Stir.

Cardamom

Cardamom is a common spice used in India related to ginger. In Ayurvedic medicine, it is often used to aid digestion and detoxify. It is good for bloating, gas, heartburn, and constipation, and it helps eliminate waste through the kidneys. We like to chew on the full pods after meals to freshen our breath.

Omega Miracle

Omega-3 fatty acids are essential to human health. While primarily found in fish, both chia and hemp seeds are good sources, too. It's a great way to start your morning instead of coffee, but you can also mix it with your coffee as a brain booster. There is evidence that coconut synergizes with chia to create better ALA conversion to DHA and EPA, but it may be not be enough for some metabolisms. Omega fats help transfer water past the cell membrane.

- 1 teaspoon ground chia seeds
- ½ cup coconut milk
- 1 tablespoon almond butter
- 1 teaspoon ground hemp seeds
- 1 teaspoon ground cinnamon
- 1 cup hot water or more, depending on your preference
- Freshly ground black pepper

Place all ingredients, except the hot water and pepper, in a blender and secure the lid. Blend for 30 to 35 seconds. Pour into a cup, add the hot water, and top with a grind of black pepper before drinking. The recipe also tastes nice with a dash of vanilla extract.

Cacao Quench for Two

The power in this nutty, chocolaty beverage is in the cacao, which is full of minerals that help activate the necessary electrical charges in our bodies.

- 1 cup fresh or frozen diced pineapple
- ¼ cup finely chopped walnuts (if you have a high-speed blender you can use whole walnuts)
- Juice of ½ lime
- 1 tablespoon coconut oil
- 1 tablespoon raw cacao powder
- 1 teaspoon maple syrup (taste test it with the sweetness of just the pineapple first)
- Pinch of coarse sea salt
- 1 cup hot water or more depending on your preference

Blend all the ingredients except the hot water and maple syrup, add the hot water, and stir well. Taste test for sweetness, and add maple syrup if desired. The salt adds depth to the flavor.

Cacao

Raw cacao powder is the least processed form of chocolate one can consume. It is grated cacao beans that came from the pods of the cacao tree. Cocoa powder is usually less expensive and is a bit more processed, but if you buy the nothing-added version—no sugar, no milk fats—it still retains many of the healthy properties of cacao powder.

Cacao powder is very rich in polyphenols, which act as antioxidants and offer strong protection against cell damage from free radicals that are formed in everyday living. It is most likely because of this that cacao has been linked to reduced mortality from cardiovascular causes and also has anti-inflammatory properties. Even the American Dietetic Association recommends a diet rich in phytochemicals, which includes dark chocolate in moderate amounts.[2]

Vegan Oat Milk with Honey, Cardamom, and Black Pepper

This is a wonderfully filling treat to drink on its own or to use as a replacement for a variety of milks. Add pepper if you want. Pepper has a long tradition of enhancing the absorption of any nutrient it's combined with as well as acting as an antimicrobial, antibacterial agent. That was why British colonials carried personal pepper grinders wherever they traveled.

MAKES ABOUT 2 QUARTS

1 cup rolled oats

6½ cups cold filtered or spring water (use 4 cups for thicker milk)

¼ cup honey

1½ teaspoons of cardamom

1 pinch sea salt

2 generous grinds of black pepper (optional)

Combine all the ingredients in a large bowl. Cover with a clean tea towel and let soak overnight at room temperature.

Use a blender or a handheld immersion blender to puree.

Strain the milk through a fine-mesh sieve into a bowl or glass jar. Refrigerate to chill, and use within 3 or 4 days.

SOUPS

Soups and broth are satisfying and a great way to hydrate, especially in the long, cold, and dry days of winter. A hand-held immersion blender makes it easy to puree soups right in the cooking pot. Try them all out; soups are fun to experiment with by adding different spices and perhaps adding another veg-etable or two. A classic time-saver is to make double batches and freeze half.

Fennel-Pistachio Soup

MAKES 4 SERVINGS

2 tablespoons ghee or unsalted butter

2 cups chopped onions

2 shallots, finely chopped

4 cups fennel (about 4 bulbs)

6 cups chicken stock

1 cup coconut milk

⅓ cup coarsely chopped pistachios

Sea salt and freshly ground pepper to taste

¼ teaspoon ground cardamom

In a large saucepan, melt the ghee over medium heat. Add the onions and shallots, and sauté, stirring frequently for 4 to 5 minutes. Add the fennel and cook for 5 minutes.

Add the stock. Simmer until the vegetables are tender, 35 to 40 minutes. Let the soup cool for 15 minutes, then puree in a blender. You may have to do this in batches, or use an immersion blender for ease.

Return the soup to the pot and whisk in the coconut milk. Reheat over medium heat before ladling into bowls and garnishing with the pistachios, salt, pepper, and cardamom.

This recipe is modified from Dr. Kara Fitzgerald's recipe to further enhance its hydrating properties.

Stracciatella

Stracciatella is the Italian version of egg drop soup. You can use store-bought stock. but this warming dish is best with homemade.

2 cups chicken or beef stock

1 large egg

¼ cup pesto

¼ cup crushed pistachios

Extra-virgin olive oil

In a pot, bring the stock to a simmer. Crack the egg into the hot stock and stir to break up the egg into noodlelike strands. Stir in the pesto.

Divide the soup between 2 bowls. Sprinkle on the pistachios and drizzle on a swirl of olive oil before serving.

Chilled Honeydew-Pear Soup

MAKES 4 SERVINGS

4 cups cubed honeydew

2 ripe pears, cored, seeded, and chopped

¾ cup coconut milk

Juice of 2 limes

1 tablespoon grated ginger

Pinch of coarse sea salt

1 teaspoon extra-virgin olive oil

Dash of ground cardamom

Place the ingredients in the blender and puree. Serve immediately or chill for several hours before dividing the soup among 4 bowls. Top each bowl with a drizzle of olive oil and a bit of cardamom. Add water, white wine, or even kombucha to adjust for the thickness you desire.

Bunny Cohen's Chicken Soup

The first thing I ever really cooked was homemade chicken soup. I made it in college by looking at the ingredients on a package of Manischewitz soup mix and replicating them using fresh ingredients. I remember discovering that it was the dill in the chicken soup that made it taste like my mom's. There is truly nothing better on a winter's day than homemade chicken soup, or "Jewish penicillin," for whatever ails you—and guess what? It's very hydrating when using real ingredients versus store-bought, fake, sodium-laden canned junk. It's actually quite easy but time consuming. Just let the soup simmer in the pot for an hour or so, checking it occasionally to see if more water is required.—Dana

> 1 small whole organic chicken (about 2½ to 3 pounds), giblets
>   discarded and chicken rinsed
> 5 to 6 carrots, cut into 2-inch pieces
> 5 to 6 stalks celery, cut into 2-inch pieces
> 1 large Spanish onion, halved
> 1 parsnip, cut into 2-inch pieces
> 1 bunch fresh dill or parsley
> Coarse sea salt and freshly ground black pepper

Put the chicken, carrots, celery, onion, parsnip, and dill in a large stock pot. Fill the pot with water, making sure the chicken is submerged. Bring to a boil, then lower the heat to a simmer. Cook for 1 hour, skimming the scum and chicken proteins from the surface every so often. Add sea salt—I like Redmond Real Salt—and some pepper to taste. Remove the chicken from the pot, but be careful not to burn yourself or, worse, let the chicken slip out of your silicone-gloved hands and fall on the floor. Put it on a plate to cool.

When the chicken is cool enough to touch, throw away the skin (or feed it to the dog), and with clean hands pull pieces of the chicken off the bone and throw it back into the soup to continue simmering for another hour. You can throw away the onion, and pull out the parsnip and mash it with butter for an easy side dish.

Bone Broth

This gets more savory as you cook it, and it also freezes well. This is a recipe is as old as the hills, as they say. Tried and true; give it a try.

MAKES 12 SERVINGS

3 pounds beef bones, such as marrow, knuckles, and oxtails with
   some meat on them, and/or chicken back, necks, and wings
1 onion, quartered
2 carrots, cut into 2-inch pieces
3 stalks celery, cut into 2-inch pieces
2 leeks, cut into 2-inch pieces
6 cloves garlic
2 tablespoons raw apple cider vinegar
3 bay leaves
2 sprigs each rosemary, parsley, and thyme
2 tablespoons black peppercorns

Heat the oven to 450°F. Place the beef bones and/or chicken pieces, onion, carrots, celery, leeks, and garlic in a roasting pan and bake for 20 minutes. Give the ingredients a toss and roast for another 10 minutes, until dark brown.

Fill a large pot with 12 cups filtered water. Add the vinegar, bay leaves, herbs, and peppercorns. Scrape the roasted bones, vegetables, and any juices into the pot. Add more water to cover as necessary.

Cover the pot and bring to a boil. Remove the lid. Reduce the heat so the broth simmers for 8 to 18 hours. Add more water to keep the ingredients submerged. The longer it simmers, the better the broth will be. Skim the occasionally to remove any foam that rises to the surface. Remove the pot from the heat. When slightly cooled, strain the broth into another container through a fine sieve and discard the bones and vegetables. Divide the broth among containers and refrigerate or freeze.

Cup-o-Broth

Sipping broths like a cup of tea shows up in all longevity cultures from Asia, through Turkey, to Italy, and now Little Italy in New York, where replacing coffee with a cup of broth in the morning is the new hip practice of foodies.

Bone Broth with Sauteed Nectarines and Pine Nuts

This savory-sweet combo is served at all Gina's parties. The following recipe is for one personal serving.

MAKES 1 SERVING

1 cup bone broth
1 nectarine
1 tablespoon ghee or unsalted butter
1 sprig rosemary
¼ cup pine nuts
Salt and pepper to taste

Gently heat bone broth in small saucepan. Thin-slice the nectarine. In a separate pan, sauté slices in ghee or butter and rosemary leaves till soft. Prepare bowl, placing pine nuts at bottom. Layer in nectarine. Pour bone broth over fruit and nuts. Remove rosemary sprig. Salt and pepper to taste.

Gazpacho

Gazpacho, a chilled soup made with raw vegetables, is accompanied with bowls of various condiments, such as hard-boiled eggs, croutons, slivered almonds, and thinly sliced scallions, so people can choose their own condiments.

MAKES 6 SERVINGS

2 pounds tomatoes, quartered
1 cucumber, peeled if not organic
1 red or green organic bell pepper, seeded
1 clove garlic
½ cup water
⅓ cup extra-virgin olive oil
2 teaspoons raw apple cider vinegar
Pinch of sea salt, black pepper, and cayenne pepper (optional)

Put all the ingredients into a blender and blend for 10 to 15 seconds. The soup should be slightly chunky, not pureed. Refrigerate until chilled. Garnish with a drizzle of olive oil. Dilute to preference with water, tomato juice, or white wine.

Tomato-Pear Gazpacho

Gazpacho should be served chilled, but not ice-cold. This version includes pears or apples. We like to sprinkle chopped pistachios on top for a bit of crunch.

MAKES 2 SERVINGS

1 medium tomato, diced, or ½ cup tomato juice

1 medium pear or apple, cut into quarters

1 tablespoon raw apple cider vinegar

1 cucumber, peeled and cut up

Juice of 1 lime

¼ cup extra-virgin olive oil

½ red bell pepper, quartered and seeded

½ to 1 cup water

1 medium clove garlic, minced

⅛ teaspoon coarse sea salt

1 small jalapeño, seeded and sliced, optional

Place all the ingredients, except for the jalapeño, in a blender and secure the lid. Blend for 10 to 15 seconds or until desired consistency is reached. The soup should be slightly chunky, not pureed. Add a slice of jalapeño, blend again, and taste for seasoning. If you want more heat, then add additional jalapeño. Refrigerate for 2 hours. If the gazpacho is too thick, stir in another ¼ to ½ cup water before serving.

Watermelon Gazpacho

Watermelon and tomatoes are a perfect combination for hydration, providing a mineral and vitamin balance between the two. And the taste will surprise you.

MAKES 4 SERVINGS

3 cups seedless watermelon pieces, plus ½ cup diced seedless
    watermelon, for garnish

2 tomatoes, quartered

1 cucumber, peeled, seeded, and cut up

1 red bell pepper, quartered and seeded

1 tablespoon extra-virgin olive oil

1 to 2 teaspoons lime juice

Pinches of sea salt, black pepper, and cayenne pepper

Put all the ingredients into a blender and blend for 10 to 15 seconds. The soup should be slightly chunky, not pureed. Taste for seasoning, adding more lime juice, salt, black pepper, and cayenne pepper as needed. Adjust to desired thickness with additional water or even white wine. Chill the gazpacho for 2 hours.

White Gazpacho

Although gazpacho is typically red, going for white or light green ingredients makes for a great summer dish.

MAKES 4 SERVINGS

4 cups honeydew melon

¾ cup coconut milk

½ cup white wine

Juice of 2 limes

2 cups diced cucumber

2 small shallots, finely sliced

2 cups green grapes, sliced

½ cup slivered almonds

Place all the ingredients, except the almonds, in a large bowl and stir well. Adjust for desired thickness by adding water. Divide into 4 bowls and garnish with the almonds. Add salt to taste.

Tip: One cup at a time, place grapes between two plastic lids, press lightly but hold firmly, and slide a sharp knife between the lids, cutting the grapes in half all in one go. You can also use this tip for cutting grape tomatoes.

SAMPLE MEALS

In the Quench Plan, it's important to have a well-rounded, nutritious diet. We offer a few great recipes to help get you going.

Breakfast

Lemon, Poppy, and Chia Pudding

You have heard of lemon poppy cake—this is even better. You're replacing a sticky carb with hydrating nutrition.

MAKES 2 SERVINGS

    2 cups coconut milk
    ½ cup whole chia seeds
    ⅓ to ¼ cup maple syrup or other sweetener
    1 tablespoon poppy seeds, or more if you like
    Juice of ½ lemon
    ½ teaspoon pure vanilla extract
    Zest of ½ lemon
    ¼ teaspoon ground cardamom
    2 pinches coarse sea salt

Mix all the ingredients together and pour into a jar or glass container and place in the refrigerator for at least 4 hours or overnight to gel. Stir or whisk a few times within the first hour to help it gel evenly.

Currant Chia Pudding

MAKES 1 SERVING

¼ cup chia seeds

1 cup light or full-fat coconut milk, depending on preference

Pinch of pink salt

2 tablespoons reduced-sugar red currant jam; any jam, such as
quince or fig, can be used

Whisk together the chia seeds and coconut milk in a bowl. Cover and refrigerate for at least 4 hours.

Top with jam before eating. You can add fresh fruit, like cubed peaches or raspberries, or a sprinkle of chopped nuts or pumpkin seeds.

Raspberry Rose Chia Jam

MAKES 1½ CUPS

10 ounces frozen raspberries

3 tablespoons rose petal jam*

3 tablespoons chia seeds

1 teaspoon cardamom

Over low heat, stir raspberries until warmed through, then add rose petal jam. Cool slightly and place in a glass storage container or jam jar; then stir in chia and cardamom. You can spread this over gluten-free bread.

You can find this in gourmet or Middle Eastern grocery stores.

Baked Avocado Nests

Avocados are 80 percent water and contain the "good" fat that our bodies need.

MAKES 4 SERVINGS

2 ripe avocados, halved and pitted
4 large eggs
4 tablespoons salsa
Fresh lime juice

Heat the oven to 425°F. Scoop out about 2 tablespoons from each avocado center to make room for egg. Place the avocados in a baking dish and crack 1 egg into the center of each avocado half. Bake for 15 to 20 minutes, until the eggs are set. Dice the remaining avocado.

Before serving, top each nest with 1 tablespoon salsa, the diced avocado, and a splash of lime juice.

Avocados

It has a pit; therefore, it's a fruit. Dana always has an avocado ripening on the windowsill. Avocados are high in the heart-healthy monounsaturated fats (like olive oil). They are full of fiber and loaded with potassium—in fact, more potassium than a banana. They also have high amounts of vitamin C, folate, and vitamin K, among other vitamins and minerals. Human studies have shown that eating avocados can lower total cholesterol, lower triglycerides, lower the bad-LDL cholesterol, and raise the good-HDL cholesterol. Last, avocados contain a lot of lutein and zeaxanthin, antioxidants important for eye health.

Lunch and Dinner

Mushroom Arugula Saute

You can use one kind of mushroom or a variety that includes button, cremini, and shiitake. Mushrooms are 98 percent water, and their fibers are famed for holding on to hydration.

MAKES 2 TO 3 SERVINGS

1 tablespoon ghee or unsalted butter

1 tablespoon extra-virgin olive oil

2 cups sliced mushrooms

3 cloves garlic, finely chopped

1 tablespoon arrowroot powder or ground chia seed or flaxseed

1 cup coconut or almond milk

4 cups arugula

1 tablespoon grainy Dijon mustard

½ teaspoon sea salt

Freshly ground black pepper

Heat the butter and olive oil in a large skillet over medium heat. Add the mushrooms and garlic and cook until the mushrooms are softened, about 10 to 12 minutes.

Add the arrowroot powder to milk and stir in with the mushrooms, cooking for 2 to 3 minutes. Stir in the arugula leaves and mustard to combine. Once the arugula is wilted, season with salt and pepper before serving hot.

Roasted Cauliflower Steak

Like many vegetables, cauliflower contains a lot of water, about 92 percent. Cauliflower becomes sweeter and caramelized when roasted. It's nothing like your mother's boiled vegetables. Serve the cauliflower accompanied by a salad of arugula, alfalfa sprouts, and sliced apples or pears.

MAKES 4 SERVINGS

1 large head cauliflower, sliced lengthwise through core 4 times
    to make 4 steaks

2 tablespoons extra-virgin olive oil

1 tablespoon raw apple cider vinegar

2 cloves garlic, minced

1 small shallot, minced

1 teaspoon rosemary leaves, minced

Coarse sea salt and freshly ground black pepper

Heat the oven to 400°F. Line a baking sheet with parchment paper. Arrange the cauliflower steaks on the lined baking sheet.

In a bowl, whisk together the olive oil, vinegar, garlic, shallot, and rosemary, then salt and pepper. Brush half of the mixture on top of the steaks. Roast the cauliflower for 15 minutes. Using a spatula, turn the cauliflower over and brush on the remaining mixture. Roast until golden, about 15 or 20 minutes.

Coconut Pineapple Iceberg Salad

Iceberg gets no respect—it has a lot of water, so it's truly hydrating. So surprise your iceberg with a tropical twist.

1 head iceberg lettuce, cut into quarters

½ cup full fat coconut milk

½ cup frozen pineapple cubes

4 tablespoons extra-virgin olive oil

1 teaspoon sherry vinegar

1 small shallot, finely diced

1 cup walnut halves

Coarse sea salt and freshly ground black pepper

Arrange the lettuce quarters on 4 salad plates. Put the coconut milk and pineapple in a blender and blend for 10 to 15 seconds. Pour the sauce over the iceberg quarters. In a small bowl, whisk the olive oil, vinegar, and shallot together. Drizzle the dressing over the lettuce wedges. Sprinkle the walnuts on top. Add salt and pepper as desired.

Triple-Threat Bean Salad

By using fresh vegetable beans, we're making sure you get the most water content, hence the name of this recipe.

MAKES 6 SERVINGS

½ pound romano beans, cut lengthwise
½ pound yellow wax beans, cut lengthwise
½ pound haricot vert, cut lengthwise
2 teaspoons shallots, minced
1 teaspoon mustard
1 teaspoon honey
¼ cup sherry vinegar
½ cup extra-virgin olive oil
1 head of radicchio or bibb lettuce

Bring a big pot of water to a boil. Add the beans and blanch for just 2 to 3 minutes. Cool in an ice bath.

To make vinaigrette, combine shallot, mustard, honey, vinegar, and olive oil. Toss beans with vinaigrette. Serve over radicchio or bibb lettuce cups.

Baked Onions

This makes a delicious summer side dish to roast chicken or turkey. Leftovers can be turned into soup by pureeing the extra cooked onions and reheating. Sprinkle with nuts like pistachios for that satisfying crunch. You may have noticed how full of water onions are. Use Spanish yellow onions in winter.

4 Vidalia onions, peeled and left whole
1 can full-fat coconut milk
4 tablespoons ghee or unsalted butter
4 sprigs fresh rosemary
1 teaspoon ground cardamom
Coarse sea salt and freshly ground black pepper

Heat oven to 350°F. Arrange the onions in a small baking dish. Pour the coconut milk over the onions. Top each onion with 1 tablespoon of ghee or butter. Tuck a sprig of rosemary around each onion. Sprinkle on the cardamom, salt, and pepper. Bake for 45 to 50 minutes, until the onions are easily pierced with a fork.

Zucchini Noodles with Pesto, Walnuts, and Olive Oil

You can make and freeze your own pesto with summer-fresh basil, but there are good commercial jars sold in supermarkets and Italian specialty stores. The great thing about these squash noodles is that everything is cooked in one pan.

MAKES 4 SERVINGS

4 medium zucchini and/or summer squash (about 2 pounds)

3 tablespoons extra-virgin olive oil

1 cup pesto

Coarse sea salt and freshly ground black pepper

1 cup chopped walnuts

Trim and spiralize the zucchini or hand-shave with a vegetable peeler.

In a skillet, heat the olive oil over medium. Add the zucchini, and cook for 5 to 7 minutes, stirring regularly, until the noodles are soft. Stir in the pesto, tossing to coat thoroughly. Season with salt and pepper.

Divide among 4 bowls and sprinkle on the walnuts and a drizzle of olive oil. Serve immediately.

Simple Roasted Chicken

Dana says, "I love this recipe because it was the first time I felt like an adult cooking this for a dinner party. And I wanted to include this recipe because—besides the fact that chicken rounds out the Quench Plan by providing great protein—everyone should know how to roast a chicken. Many young adults living on their own for the first time don't know how. We've lost some tried-and-true cooking skills, and I think we need to bring it back to our kitchens."

MAKES 4 SERVINGS

1 3-pound organic roasting chicken, giblets discarded and
    chicken rinsed

Coarse sea salt and freshly ground black pepper

1 cup shallots, roughly cut

1 lemon, halved

2 rosemary sprigs

2 tablespoons (¼ stick) butter, melted

Preheat over to 425°F. Season chicken inside and out with salt and pepper. Stuff with rough-cut shallots, lemon, and rosemary sprigs. Coat with butter.

Roast on rack for 15 minutes. Turn oven down to 350°F. Cook for another 30 to 45 minutes. (You can check the internal temperature—you'll want a minimum of 165°F—by placing a thermometer in the thickest muscle, typically the thigh.)

Let rest for 20 minutes, and enjoy!

Broiled Fish

This is another basic "grown-up" recipe—and it also provides great protein to supplement the Quench Plan.

> 1 whole fish such as branzino, porgy, or trout (cleaned, scaled, gutted, and trimmed of the fins, leaving only the head and tail in place), about 1½ pounds
> ⅓ cup plus 1 tablespoon olive oil
> Salt and pepper
> 2 tablespoons dried oregano, divided
> 2 lemons
> ⅓ cup extra-virgin olive oil

Preheat the broiler. Adjust the oven rack to the upper third of the oven. Rub both sides of fish with olive oil, then season with salt, pepper, and 1 tablespoon of dried oregano. Make sure to season the cavity as well.

Broil with the fish as close to the heat source as possible until the skin is crispy—about 7 minutes—then flip the fish and broil the other side until crispy.

In a mason jar, combine the juice of 2 lemons with ⅓ cup extra-virgin olive oil, 1 tablespoon dried oregano, and salt and pepper. Shake vigorously. Pour over the fish. Garnish with lemon slices, serve, and eat!

Desserts

Why shouldn't desserts be hydrating? Ours are designed to send you out the door without that dragged-out, dried-up feeling.

Coconut Lavender Panna Cotta with Black Peppercorns

This recipe has its origins in medieval times. Ours is a variation on one that would have been served at a wedding to Italian royalty...and oh, yeah, it is superhydrating, too.

MAKES 4 SERVINGS

- 1 13.5-ounce can full-fat coconut milk, divided
- 1¼ teaspoons grass-fed gelatin or collagen powder, such as Great Lakes brand
- 1 teaspoon vanilla extract
- ⅓ cup maple syrup
- 4 drops lavender extract
- A grind of black peppercorns to top each bowl

In a small saucepan, whisk together 1 cup of the coconut milk with the powdered gelatin. Allow to sit for 5 minutes, to allow the gelatin to "bloom." Add in the vanilla and lavender extract then gently heat the mixture over medium-low heat, whisking well to help the gelatin dissolve. Be careful *not* to boil this mixture! Once the gelatin has completely dissolved, remove from the heat and stir in the maple syrup and remaining coconut milk.

Pour the mixture into four 6-ounce ramekins. Cover and refrigerate until set, for at least 4 hours. Serve with a fresh grind of black pepper.

Frozen Grapes

One of the best treats we can recommend for a cooling and hydrating snack or dessert are frozen seedless green grapes. Freeze a bunch of grapes in plastic bags and they'll be ready to enjoy.

Popsicles

Who says popsicles are just for hot summer days? These cool, soothing treats can be made ahead and enjoyed for breakfast, snacks, or dessert. Use any kind of frozen berries or fruit. We recommend using more powerful blenders for our popsicle recipes. Some of our popsicle recipes can be used as sorbets straight from the blender. In these recipes, each individual popsicle is about 4 ounces.

Raspberry Popsicles

MAKES 6 POPSICLES

2 tablespoons chia seeds
5 ounces coconut milk, divided
1 cup fresh or frozen raspberries
4 tablespoons honey
Juice of 1 lime

In a small bowl, soak the chia seeds in 1 ounce of coconut milk for 5 to 10 minutes. Put the chia seeds, remaining coconut milk, raspberries, honey, and lime juice into a blender and puree. Divide the mixture among 6 bisphenol A (BPA)–free popsicle molds and freeze until solid.

Chocolate-Avocado Popsicles

MAKES 6 POPSICLES

3 small ripened avocados, peeled, pitted, and cut up

1 13.5-ounce can coconut milk

6 tablespoons honey

½ cup cocoa powder

Pinch of sea salt

1 teaspoon pure vanilla extract

1 teaspoon coconut oil

Put all the ingredients into a blender and puree. Divide the mixture among 6 BPA-free popsicle molds and freeze until solid.

Creamy Banana-Cashew Popsicles

MAKES 6 POPSICLES

2 cups raw unsalted cashews

1 cup coconut milk

2 bananas

2 tablespoons honey

½ cup fresh or frozen blueberries or pitted cherries

2 teaspoons pure vanilla extract

Put the cashews in a bowl, cover with water, and soak for 2 to 6 hours, until soft, then drain.

Put all the ingredients into a blender and puree. Divide the mixture among 6 BPA-free popsicle molds and freeze until solid.

Orange Popsicles

1½ cups fresh orange juice

1 cup coconut milk

2 tablespoons fresh lemon juice

2 tablespoons honey (optional)

Put all the ingredients into a blender and puree. Divide the mixture among 6 BPA-free popsicle molds and freeze until solid.

Berry-Lavender Popsicles

MAKES 6 POPSICLES

1 cup fresh or frozen blueberries

1 cup fresh or frozen blackberries

1 banana

¾ cup coconut milk or cashew milk

¼ cup coconut butter (pureed coconut, not oil)

2 tablespoons honey

4 drops lavender extract

1 teaspoon pure vanilla extract

Pinch of pink or coarse sea salt

Reserve ¼ cup each of the blueberries and blackberries and divide them among 6 BPA-free popsicle molds. Put all the remaining ingredients into a blender and puree. Pour the mixture into the molds and freeze until solid.

Coconut-Lime Avocado Popsicles

MAKES 6-8 POPSICLES

1 13.5-ounce can coconut milk

2 small ripened avocados, pitted and peeled

½ cup fresh lime juice

¼ cup coconut water

¼ cup honey

1 tablespoon lemon zest

Put all the ingredients into a blender and puree. Divide the mixture among 6 BPA-free popsicle molds and freeze until solid.

Afterword

You Are a Body of Water

With *Quench*, we set before you a number of powerful arguments for making hydration a first priority for you, with new ways to do it. You now know the eight-glasses-a-day advice may not be best in our water-challenged world. Water is not only blue; you can get it better from green. In a time when we are thirsty for new knowledge, we wanted to show not only how hydration works but how science works.

From Dr. Pollack's amazing experiments showing a new phase of water, to the discovery of fascia as a true water system running throughout our body, it seems we are only just beginning to understand the connection between water and our own bodies. Dr. Jean-Claude Guimberteau's video of fascia pushed us to the conclusion that fascia is not only an inner irrigation system but an electrical and information system, driven by water energy.

Other ground-shifting science was critical to the forming of Quench, some of it breaking even as we were writing. Two more important findings came from Dr. Pollack. He proved that light waves charge water molecules with energy, and he confirmed that gel water was found in all plant cells. Now water, water, is everywhere you see green.

The *Journal of Cell Science* published Yi-Wen Xu's paper,

showing green plants can harvest light *inside* of us to release cus-
tomized nutrients, another ground-shifting study we are only
beginning to understand. And all this new science is unfolding
right in the midst of the microbiome revolution. Whatever is
happening to us is happening to our bacteria, too. And then Dr.
Maiken Nedergaard reported that there was an entire drainage
system in our brains no one had seen before. Water in our bodies
is at the very frontier of science, in your time.

So never again think of water as a mere something to wash
down our supper or our pills, or to guzzle after a long run. Water
should be what we go for first thing in the morning, it's how we
get through the day, and it's how we cleanse our brain at night.

You're primed now to know that the first question you should
ask yourself when you are feeling off—whether it be fatigue,
brain fog, or pain somewhere—is "Am I hydrated enough?"
Why? Because you, too, along with this planet, are a body of
water. Ninety-nine percent of you.

Acknowledgments

Dana's Acknowledgments

With the deepest gratitude I would like to acknowledge some very special people, all of whom in one way or another made the process of writing this book possible.

First I must thank Gina Bria, my coauthor, whom I have grown to know and love; thank you for bringing me that delicious smoothie that fateful day almost three years ago. My agent, Linda Loewenthal, thank you for not only having my back but for your wonderful editorial contributions. To Michelle Howry, my editor at Hachette, thank you for your guidance. Thank you for your contributions and editing, Kathy Huck, Camille Pagan, and Leslie Meredith.

For my patients, I am thankful for you each and every day for allowing me into your lives and giving me back so much more than I can ever express. You are the purpose in my life.

For my friends, thank you for your support and encouragement. They say you are lucky if you have one best friend—then I am beyond blessed, as I have four: Patricia Richardson, Liz Belson, Leslie Dick, and Susan Lazarus. For their assistance and reassurance, Steve Feldman, Devon Nola, Brooke Freeman, Michael Sherman, Sam Carter, and Manju Moreno. For keeping me sane and healthy, thank you to Dr. Daniel Fenster and the whole staff at Complete Wellness: Jan Stritzler, Denise Lucero,

Stefani Lipani, Dr. Shilo Kramer, Dr. Dan Kay, Masae Shimo-moto, Dr. David Hashemipour, and Tim Coyle.

For my family, who lift me up, particularly Lisa Albury, Jeff Cohen, and Randi Henry. I am so proud to be a part of our crazy family. And I can't forget my other crazy family members: Jamie Camche, Aunt Patsy, Uncle Buddy, and Viola and Michelle Gulinello. Thank you for your love and praises—they keep me going and raise me up every day. I love you all and your own crazy families—my extended family.

And especially Henry Caplan: Thank you for your love and support and notably for your goofiness. You add the color to my world, yet you also add the sanity and calm when I most need it. I love you very much.

Gina's Acknowledgments

Authors' confession: We didn't really write this book; it wrote *us*. We just were willing to put it to page, but over and over again new information would *find us*. Who do you acknowledge under those conditions? Some stranger in a bank line would begin explaining a massage technique and it was relevant. It would go right in the book. So many new studies came in, often published just weeks before our manuscript was due. We'd get e-mails from organizations we'd never heard of with break-through reports. It was like a cosmic assignment lasering down on us to get this information out there. You are part of this, too, so please pass it on! We believe it is so important to rethink our water use for all us bodies of water, whether humans, animals, plants, bathtubs, sinks, water bottles, wading pools, streams, rivers, lakes, even the little body of a raindrop. Join us in our further work to be blessed by water and bless it back. Share your hydration stories with us at www.hydrationfoundation.org.

Among my colleagues, I offer acknowledgement to Dana Cohen, MD. "Let's write a book." was the inspired moment. I must and want to acknowledge Dr. Gerald Pollack, a gentleman scientist and a most generous champion for water. His life's work is the genesis of *Quench*. Linda Loewenthal, agent extraordinaire, who brought *Quench* into publishing reality. She never even once thought it wasn't going to happen. Michelle Howry, our editor at Hachette Book Group, whose joy in this project was our open door. Mary Ellen O'Neill, who has been personally editing my life for more than twenty-five years. Judith Kunst, prescient editor, who knew what the reader wanted before we even wrote the book. For early help with the manuscript, thanks to Tamar Grimm, who can read a book by putting her hand on it, and Erin Inclan, who can get anybody to read anything. The Metropolitan Museum of Art at the Cloisters and Michael Carter, the librarian there, gave generous access to their rare collection of botanical and herbal manuscripts. To Brother Ezekial Brennan and the twelve Benedictine monks at the Monastery of the Holy Cross in Chicago, who provided a six-day writing retreat in silence...and singing. Ani Barnes, director of physical conditioning at Columbia University, who first taught me to "move like an elegant horse" and inspired my research on hydration and movement. Karen Balliett, Sunny Bates, Anita Cooney, and Margo Fish, each, in their unique way, a Water Queen. They allowed themselves to be experimented upon for the sake of adventurous science. Amy Cherry, founder of Shou Sugi Ban House Spa in the Hamptons, New York, for supporting research on hydrotherapies. Christina Marie Kimball and her husband, Alex, for providing a "water thought retreat" on their boat, *Gypsy Wind*, which set my course for becoming as much a body as possible before death. Ellie Costa and Max Frye, for the kind loan of their house in Woods Hole, Massachusetts, for an eight-day writing retreat. This led to two seredipitious encounters at the Marine Biological Laboratory, based in Woods Hole, that confirmed our *Quench* research. In that eight-day stretch I met Dr. Rudolf Oldenbourg, director of the Cellular Dynamics Program at the MBL. Before my very eyes, he actually stretched simple plastic wrap under a high-speed microscope, and I watched how the two central principles in our book, *light waves* and *stretching,* aligned the molecules for more efficient function. Dr. Lora Hooper, chair of the Immunology Department at University of Texas Southwestern Medical Center, was also and equally serendipitously in Woods Hole for one night only. She was there to deliver the famed Friday Evening Lecture, and almost the entire science community at MBL showed up to hear her. Her presentation demonstrated how all cells, and also all bacteria, have molecular clocks requiring light. Laura Hames Franklin shared anatomical and movement training and inspirational support and information for *Quench.* TEDxNewYork Salon Bodies of Water supporters, Jennifer Phillips, Diana Ayton-Shenker, Grandmother Elder Nancy Audry, and Victoria Cummings have provided access to Native American water wisdom traditions. Thanks to my teacher, David Crow, herbal master and founder of Floracopea, who catapulted me to a new understanding of plants as our biological allies: our evolutionary partners with their own intelligent solutions to our common environmental challenges.

And of course, my family, God help them: James Vescovi, my husband, and my offspring, Alma, Luca, and Carlo, but special acknowledgements to my sister, Gretchen, who has never failed to inspire and support me, and whose special care of our mother, Stephanie, taught and blessed me.

Appendix

Allergy Elimination Diet

The elimination diet described on the following pages is a modification of a diet recommended by William Crook, MD, a pioneer in the evaluation and management of hidden food allergies.[1] The purpose of this diet is to identify hidden food allergens that may be causing some or all of your symptoms. During the elimination period, all common allergens are completely eliminated from the diet for two to three weeks. After your symptoms improve, foods are added back one at a time, to determine which foods have been causing symptoms.

FOODS YOU MUST AVOID

Dairy products: Milk, cheese, butter, yogurt, sour cream, cottage cheese, whey, casein, sodium caseinate, calcium caseinate, and any food containing these.

Wheat: Most breads, spaghetti, noodles, pasta, most flour, baked goods, durum semolina, farina, and many gravies. Although this diet prohibits wheat, it is not a gluten-free diet. Oats, barley, and rye are allowed.

Corn: Whole corn and foods made with corn (such as corn chips, tortillas, popcorn, and breads, and other baked goods that list corn as an ingredient). Also avoid products that contain corn oil, vegetable oil from an unspecified source, corn syrup, corn sweetener, dextrose, and glucose.

Eggs: Whites and yolks, and any product that contains eggs.

Citrus fruits: Oranges, grapefruits, lemons, limes, tangerines, and foods that contain citrus fruits.

Coffee, tea, and alcohol: Avoid both caffeinated and decaffeinated coffee, as well as standard (such as Lipton) tea and decaffeinated tea. Herb teas are allowed, except those that contain citrus.

Refined sugars: Avoid table sugar and any foods that contain it, such as candy, soft drinks, pies, cake, cookies, chocolate, sweetened applesauce, and so on. Other names for sugar include sucrose, high-fructose corn syrup, corn syrup, corn sweetener, fructose, cane juice, glucose, dextrose, maltose, maltodextrin, and levulose. These must all be avoided. Some patients (depending on their suspected sensitivity to refined sugar) will be allowed one to three teaspoons per day of pure, unprocessed honey, maple syrup, or barley malt syrup. This will be decided on an individual basis. Patients restricted from all sugars should not eat dried fruit. Those who are not restricted from all sugars may eat unsulfured (organically grown) dried fruits sparingly. Because little is known about alternative sweeteners such as stevia, they should not be used during the elimination phase.

Food additives: Avoid artificial colors, flavors, preservatives, texturing agents, artificial sweeteners, and so on. Most diet sodas and other dietetic foods contain artificial ingredients and must be avoided. Grapes, prunes, and raisins that are not organically grown may contain sulfites and should be avoided.

Any other food you eat three times a week or more should be avoided and tested later.

Known allergens: Avoid any food you know you are allergic to, even if it is allowed on this diet.

Tap water (including cooking water): Tap water is eliminated in cases where more extreme sensitivity is suspected. If tap water is not allowed, use spring or distilled water bottled in glass or hard plastic. Soft (collapsible) plastic containers tend to leach plastic into the water, so avoid water bottled in those. Bottles with the numbers 3 or 7 are likely to leach phthalates. Choose bottles and containers that are free of BPA. Some water filtration systems do not take out all potential allergens. Take your water with you, including to work and to restaurants.

Read labels

Hidden allergens are frequently found in packaged foods. "Flour" usually means wheat, "vegetable oil" may mean corn oil, and casein and whey are dairy products. Make sure your vitamins are free of wheat, corn, sugar, citrus, yeast, and artificial colorings.

FOODS YOU MAY EAT

Cereals: *Hot*—oatmeal, oat bran, cream of rye, Arrowhead Mills Rice and Shine. *Dry*—Barbara's or Erewhon's puffed rice, Barbara's Brown Rice Crisps cereal. Diluted apple juice with apple slices and nuts go well on cereal. You may use soy milk that has no corn oil or sugar added (such as some Eden Soy and Rice Dream products). Most of these foods are available in health food stores and some grocery stores.

Grains and flour products: *Flours*—soy, rice, potato,

buckwheat, and bean flours. *Breads*—rice, 100 percent rye, spelt, or millet bread (as long as they do not contain dairy, eggs, sugar, or wheat). *Cooked whole grains*—oats, millet, barley, buckwheat groats (kasha), brown rice, brown rice pasta, rice macaroni, spelt (flour and pasta), amaranth, and quinoa. *Other*—100 percent rice cakes (such as Quaker), rice crackers, rye crackers, Orgran Buckwheat Gluten-Free Crispbread, flax crackers (from Foods Alive), Blue Dragon Spring Roll Wrappers, Oriental noodles (such as 100 percent buckwheat Soba noodles from Eden), and Ka-Me Bean Threads. Most of these products are available at health food stores and can be ordered from any grocery store that carries Arrowhead Mills, Bob's Red Mill, Shilo Farms, or Ancient Harvest.

Legumes: Soybeans, tofu, lentils, peas, chickpeas, navy beans, kidney beans, black beans, string beans, and others. Dried beans should be soaked overnight. Pour off the water and rinse before cooking. Canned beans often contain added sugar or other potential allergens. Some cooked beans packaged in glass jars (generally sold at health food stores) contain no sugar. You may also use bean dips (like hummus) that do not contain sugar, lemon, or additives. Canned soups such as split pea, lentil, and turkey/vegetable (without additives) may also be used. Companies that make acceptable products include Amy's, Kettle Cuisine, and Imagine Foods.

Vegetables and fruits: Use a wide variety. All vegetables except corn and all fruits except citrus are permitted.

Proteins: Beef, lamb, pork, chicken, turkey, and fish. Lamb rarely causes allergic reactions and can be used by most people who have multiple sensitivities. Grain/bean casseroles may be used as an alternative to animal foods (see vegetarian cookbooks for recipes). Shrimp and most canned or packaged shellfish (such as lobster, crab, and oysters) may contain sulfites and should be avoided. Canned tuna, salmon, and other canned fish are allowed.

Nuts and seeds: Nuts may be eaten raw or roasted (without sugar) To prevent rancidity, nuts and seeds should be kept in an airtight container in the refrigerator. You may also use nut butters (such as peanut butter, almond butter, cashew butter, walnut butter, sesame butter, hemp seed butter, and sesame tahini). Companies that make acceptable products include Full Circle, Arrowhead Mills, and Natalie's. Nut butters go well on celery sticks and crackers. In recipes, freshly ground flaxseed can be used instead of egg. One tablespoon of ground flaxseed with ⅓ cup of water will bind in recipes as well as one egg, but additional leavening may be needed depending on the recipe.

Oils and fats: Sunflower, safflower, olive, sesame, peanut, flaxseed, canola, and soy oils may be used. Do not use corn oil or vegetable oil from an unspecified source (which is usually corn oil). Soy, sunflower, and safflower margarines are acceptable from an allergy standpoint, but most margarines contain trans fatty acids (which may promote heart disease) and are therefore not recommended. Vegetable spreads and bean spreads (such as hummus) may be used instead of butter or margarine. Ripe avocado can also be spread on sandwiches in place of mayonnaise.

Snacks: Any permitted food can be eaten as a snack any time of day. Acceptable snacks include Danielle Veggie Chips and Gorge Delights's Just Fruit Bars. Other good snacks include celery, carrot sticks, and other vegetables; fruit (no citrus); and unsalted fresh nuts and seeds.

Beverages: Acceptable drinks include spring water in glass bottles or hard plastic, herb teas (no lemon or orange), non–citrus fruit juices without sugar or additives (dilute 50:50 with water), and soy or rice milk without corn oil (such as Eden Soy Plain or Rice Dream Original). Cafix, Inka, and Kaffree Roma may be used as coffee substitutes. Tap water contains chlorine, fluoride, and other potentially allergenic chemicals. In some cases, spring water in glass or hard plastic bottles is the only water allowed. This would include water used for cooking. If tap water is eliminated, it should be reintroduced as if it were a test food. Restrictions on the type of water permitted will be made on a case-by-case basis.

Thickeners: Rice, oat, millet, barley, soy, or amaranth flours; arrowroot powder; agar flakes; and kudzu powder may be used as thickeners.

Spices and condiments: Acceptable items include salt (in moderation), pepper, herbal spices (without preservatives, citrus, or sugar), garlic, ginger, onions, catsup, and mustard without sugar (such as catsup from Muir Glen and mustard from Full Circle), Bragg Liquid Aminos (as a replacement for soy sauces that contain wheat or additives), and vitamin C crystals in water (as a substitute for lemon juice).

Miscellaneous foods: Sugar-free spaghetti sauce (such as Amy's) and fruit jellies without sugar or citrus (such as Suzanne's fruit spreads).

GENERAL SUGGESTIONS

Do not restrict calories. Start with a good breakfast, eat frequently throughout the day, and consume at least four glasses of water per day. If you do not eat enough, you may experience symptoms of low blood sugar, such as fatigue, irritability, headache, and rapid weight loss. Eat a wide variety of foods. Do not rely on just a few foods, because you may become allergic to foods you eat every day. To ensure adequate fiber intake, eat beans, permitted whole grains, whole fruits and vegetables, homemade vegetable soup, nuts, and seeds. Be sure to chew thoroughly, in order to enhance digestion.

Plan your meals. Plan your meals for the entire week. Take some time before starting the diet in order to develop meal plans, and stock the kitchen with adequate amounts of permitted foods. For ideas, look through cookbooks that specialize in hypoallergenic diets. Most meals can be modified easily to meet the requirements of the diet, without changing the meal plan for the rest of your family. When you go to the health food store, ask for assistance in locating appropriate breads, crackers, cereals, soups, and so on. Some people find it useful to prepare additional foods on the weekend, which helps to cut down on thinking and preparation time during the week. If you need further assistance or ideas, talk with your diet counselor at the doctor's office.

Use the Internet. For people with limited access to a health food store, searching for hypoallergenic foods on one of the Internet sites listed below can be helpful. Perform the search as an "advanced search," specifying as many terms as the site allows, such as *wheat free, corn free, dairy free, casein free,* and *no added sugar.* This type of search eliminates many of the unacceptable products, but you will still need to read the ingredients of products that interest you. You can buy directly from websites such as Glutenfreemall.com or special-order the foods through your local grocery.

Dine out. Do not hesitate to ask questions or make requests. For example, you could ask for fish topped with slivered almonds, cooked without added seasoning, butter, or lemon. Get a baked potato with a slice of onion on top. Order steak or lamb chops with fresh vegetables, also prepared without added seasonings (with the exception of garlic and plain herbs). Make sure the salad bar does not use sulfites as a preservative, and bring your own dressing (oil and cider vinegar with chopped nuts/ seeds and fresh herbs). Carry pure water, snacks, seasonings, and so on wherever you go, to supplement your meals or to have something on hand if you get hungry.

Withdrawal symptoms. About one in four patients develops mild withdrawal symptoms within a few days of starting the diet. Withdrawal symptoms may include fatigue, irritability, headaches, malaise, or increased hunger. These symptoms generally disappear within two to five days and are usually followed by an improvement in your original symptoms. If withdrawal symptoms are too uncomfortable, take buffered vitamin C (sodium ascorbate or calcium ascorbate) at a dose of 1,000 mg in tablet or capsule form or ¼ teaspoon of the crystals, up to four times per day. Your doctor may also prescribe alkali salts (a mixture of sodium bicarbonate and potassium bicarbonate, taken as needed at a dose of ¼ to ½ teaspoon dissolved in six to eight ounces of water up to three to four times per day). In most cases, withdrawal symptoms are not severe and do not require treatment. When starting the elimination diet, it is best to discontinue all the foods abruptly (cold turkey), rather than easing into the diet slowly.

TESTING INDIVIDUAL FOODS

It usually takes two to three weeks for symptoms to improve enough to allow you to retest foods. However, you may begin retesting sooner if you have been feeling a lot better for at least five days and have been on the diet for at least ten days. If you have been on the diet for four weeks and feel no better, contact your doctor's office for further instructions. Most patients do improve. Some feel so much better on the diet that they decide not to test the foods. This could be a mistake. If you wait too long to retest, your allergies may settle down and you will not be able to provoke symptoms by food testing. As a result, you will not know which foods you are allergic to. If reintroducing certain foods causes a recurrence of symptoms, you are probably allergic to those foods.

Food Sources for Testing

Test pure sources of the various foods. For example, do not use pizza to test cheese, because pizza also contains wheat and possibly corn oil. Do not use bread to test wheat, because bread often contains other potential allergens. It is best to use organic foods when testing, so as not to risk interference from pesticides, hormones, or other additives that may be present in some foods.

Testing Procedure

Test one new food each day. If your main symptom is arthritic pain, test one new food every other day. Allergic reactions to test foods usually occur within ten minutes to twelve hours after ingestion. However, joint pains may be delayed by as much as forty-eight hours. Eat a relatively large amount of each test food. For example, on the day you test milk, consume a large glass at breakfast, along with any of the other foods on the "permitted" list. If, after one serving, your original symptoms come back or if you develop a headache, bloating, nausea, dizziness, or fatigue, then do not eat that food again and place it on your "allergic" list. If no symptoms occur, eat the food again for lunch and dinner and watch for reactions. Even if the food is well tolerated, do not add it back into your diet until you have finished testing all of the foods. If you do experience a reaction, wait until your symptoms have improved before testing the next food. In some instances, it may not be clear whether the symptoms you are experiencing are due to the most recently eaten food or to a delayed reaction to a previously eaten food. If you are uncertain whether you have reacted to a particular food, remove it from your diet and retest it four to five days later. You do not have to test foods you never eat.

Do not test foods you already know cause symptoms.

Foods may be tested in any order. Begin testing on a day you are feeling well. Keep a daily journal that records individual food challenges and symptoms.

Food Testing

Dairy tests

Test milk and cheese on separate days. You may wish to test several cheeses on different days, since some people are allergic to certain cheeses but not to others. It is usually not necessary to test yogurt, cottage cheese, or butter separately.

Wheat test

Use Wheatena (with no milk or sugar) or another pure wheat cereal. You may add soy or rice milk.

Corn test

Use fresh ears of corn or frozen corn (without sauces or preservatives).

Egg test

Test the whites and yolks on separate days, using hard-boiled eggs.

Citrus test

Test oranges, grapefruits, lemons, and limes individually on separate days. The lemon and lime can be squeezed into water. For oranges and grapefruits, use whole, fresh fruit.

Tap water and frequently eaten foods

Test tap water, if you have eliminated it. Also test the foods you have eliminated because they had been eaten frequently.

Optional tests

If any of the following items are not now a part of your diet, or if you are committed to eliminating them from your diet, there is no need to test them. However, if you have been consuming any of these items regularly, it is a good idea to test them and find out how they affect you. Reactions to these foods and beverages may be severe in some cases. They should be tested only on days that you can afford to feel bad.

Coffee and tea: Test on separate days. Do not add milk, nondairy creamer, or sugar. But an acceptable soy or rice milk may be added. If you use decaffeinated coffee, test it separately. Coffee, tea, decaffeinated coffee, and decaffeinated tea are separate tests.

Sugar: Put four teaspoons of cane sugar in a drink or on cereal, or mix it with another food.

Chocolate: Use one to two tablespoons of pure baker's chocolate or Hershey's cocoa powder.

Food additives: Buy a set of McCormick or French's food dyes and colors. Put ½ teaspoon of each color in a glass. Add one teaspoon of the mixture to a glass of water and drink. If you wish, you may test each color separately.

Alcohol: Beer, wine, and hard liquor may require testing on different days, since the reactions to each may be different. Have two drinks per test day, but only if you can afford not to feel well that day and possibly the next day.

After the testing

After the testing is finished, please return to your doctor's office for a follow-up visit. Bring your journal with you, in order to review your experiences with the doctor.

Suggestions for Self-Help

If you have an allergic constitution and eat the same foods every day, you may eventually become allergic to those foods. After you have discovered which foods you can eat safely, make an attempt to rotate your diet. A four-day schedule is necessary for some highly allergic people, but most people can tolerate foods more frequently than every four days. You may eventually be able to tolerate allergenic foods, after you have avoided them for six to twelve months.

However, if you continue to eat these foods more frequently than every fourth day, the allergy may return.

Consume a wide variety of foods, not just a few favorites. If you are rotating foods, be sure to avoid all forms of the food when you are on an "off" day. For example, if you are rotating corn, avoid corn chips, corn oil, corn sweeteners, and so on, except on the days you are eating corn and corn products. It is not necessary to do strict food rotation during the elimination and retesting periods.

Watch for other allergic reactions. If you have an allergic constitution, you may be allergic to foods other than those you have eliminated and tested on this diet. Pay attention to what you are eating, and review recent meals if you develop symptoms. You can then eliminate that food for two weeks and test it again, to see if it triggers the same symptoms.

You can also visit https://doctorgaby.com for more information.

Resources

AUTHORS' WEBSITES

- www.drdanacohen.com
- www.completewellnessnyc.com
- www.hydrationfoundation.org

BOOKS AND ARTICLES WORTH YOUR TIME

- As we mentioned in our preface, this book greatly influenced us when we were first thinking about writing *Quench*: Dr. Fereydoon Batmanghelidj's *Your Body's Many Cries for Water* (Global Health Solutions, 2008).
- A must-read book is by Dr. Gerald Pollack written for a lay audience, and easily digestible, with cartoons, no less, on gel water and its use for energy in the body: *The Fourth Phase of Water: Beyond Solid, Liquid, and Vapor* (Ebner and Sons, 2013).
- "The Fourth Phase of Water: Implications for Energy and Health," published in the Winter 2015 issue of *Wise Traditions* (volume 16, no. 4) by Gerald Pollack.
- In an informative blog called "Water, Energy, and the Perils of Dehydration," the late Nicholas Gonzalez, MD, discusses the groundbreaking book *Your Body's Many Cries for*

Water by Dr. Batmanghelidj and the epidemic of chronic dehydration. You can find it at https://www.greenmed info.com/blog/water-energy-and-perils-dehydration.

- The study "Water, Hydration and Health" by Dr. Barry Popkin et al. is a great read for a deep dive into water and health (*Nutrition Reviews*, volume 68, no. 8, August 2010, pages 439–458).

- An important book that explores our relationship with water is M. J. Pangman and Melanie Evans's *Dancing with Water: The New Science of Water* (Uplifting Press, 2011).

- If you want to know more about fat's role in our bodies, look no further than *Know Your Fats: The Complete Primer for Understanding the Nutrition of Fats, Oils, and Cholesterol* by Mary G. Enig, PhD (Bethesda Press, 2000).

- For exercises that are best for women, take a look at *Strength Training Exercises for Women* by Joan Pagano (DK Publishing, 2013).

- If you want to read up on just how exercise can affect the brain, read *Spark: The Revolutionary New Science of Exercise and the Brain* by John Ratey, MD (Little, Brown, 2008).

- Teresa Tapp's *Fit and Fabulous in 15 Minutes* (Ballantine, 2006) is a great place to start if you are looking for a go-to resource on fascia stretching and getting into shape quickly and easily.

- Mary Bond's *The New Rules of Posture: How to Sit, Stand, and Move in the Modern World* (Healing Arts Press, 2006) is a great resource for good posture.

- For further study on the Egoscue Method, to straight to the source with *The Egoscue Method of Health Through Motion* by Pete Egoscue with Roger Gittines (William Morrow, 1993).

- Another great resource for exercise techniques is Eric Franklin's *Franklin Method: Ball and Imagery Exercises for*

Relaxed and Flexible Shoulders, Neck and Thorax (Orthope-dic Physical Therapy Products, 2008).

- Read Roger Jahnke's *The Healer Within: Using Traditional Chinese Techniques to Release Your Body's Own Medicine, Movement, Massage, Meditation, Breathing* (HarperOne, 1998) for great Eastern practices of movement meditations and breathe and stress reduction.

- To learn more about hydration and breathing, read Patrick McKeown's *Close Your Mouth: Buteyko Clinic Handbook for Perfect Health* (Buteyko Books, 2005).

NUTRITION AND WELLNESS SOURCES: SHOPPING WEBSITES

- **https://www.costco.com:** Costco is a surprising resource of some good organic produce and products, like organic virgin coconut oil.

- **https://www.grownyc.org:** This sustainability resource for New Yorkers (our neck of the woods) includes local farmers' markets and recycling information.

- **http://www.localfarmmarkets.org:** Search nationwide for farmers' markets.

- **https://www.knowfoods.com:** This site offers delicious low glycemic, grain-free, gluten-free, dairy-free, peanut-free, soy-free, and yeast-free products. No kidding.

- **https://www.mountainroseherbs.com:** This is a good source of bulk herbs and spices.

- **https://www.thrivemarket.com:** Organic products at good prices are sold here.

MUST-WATCH VIDEOS AND TEDX TALKS

- Dr. Jean-Claude Guimberteau's groundbreaking video of fascia (in French): https://www.youtube.com/watch?v=eW0lvOVKDxE
- An excellent explanation of Dr. Guimberteau's findings by *Functional Therapy Magazine*: https://www.youtube.com/watch?v=qSXpX4wyoY8
- Dr. Gerald Pollack's TEDx talk, "Water, Cells, Life," on the fourth phase of water: https://www.youtube.com/watch?v=p9UC0chfXcg
- TEDx New York Salon's "Bodies of Water Conference" video: https://www.hydrationfoundation.org/copy-of-highlights-1
- Dr. Stephanie Seneff's TEDx Talk, "The Mineral Power for Your Body's Electrical Supply": https://www.youtube.com/watch?v=fDWEVXhaydc
- Gina Bria's TEDx Talk, "How to Grow Water: It's Not Only Blue, It's Green": https://www.youtube.com/watch?v=kAiCeRZLCoE
- Gillian Ferrabee's TEDx Talk "Water as a Conductor for Creative Flow": https://www.youtube.com/watch?v=ryYTxm7k7mg
- Dr. Adam Wexler's TEDx Talk, "The Bridge Between Water and Life": https://www.youtube.com/watch?v=hPM1l93mGZw
- Amy Cuddy's TED Talk, "Your Body Language May Shape Who You Are": https://www.youtube.com/watch?v=Ks-_Mh1QhMc
- Master Tiong's Facial Detox Self-Massage Technique: https://www.youtube.com/watch?v=p5p9AzC9LE8

ONLINE NUTRITION AND MOVEMENT RESOURCES

- **https://www.beautifulonraw.com:** Tonya Zavasta gives a modern-day twist on ancient Russian and Ukrainian skin and health techniques.
- **https://blog.bulletproof.com:** David Asprey is a famed biohacker who experiments on his own body and passes the word along. He originated the new global craze for putting fats in coffee, called Bulletproof Coffee.
- **https://www.eldoamethod.com:** Dr. Guy Voyer's ELDOA Method offers excellent stretch routines.
- **http://www.egoscue.com:** Peter Egoscue's method for ending chronic pain is among the most simple and straightforward of movement techniques.
- **http://www.floracopeia.com:** David Crow, a master herbalist, provides products and tips for hydrating with aromatherapies.
- **https://www.drkarafitzgerald.com:** Dr. Kara Fitzgerald has a doctorate in naturopathic medicine. Her website provides many hydrating recipes.
- **https://www.foundmyfitness.com:** Dr. Rhonda Patrick reviews latest science findings on health.
- **https://www.laurahamesfranklin.com:** Laura Hames Franklin offers anatomy lessons through visualization and a unique body-training program.
- **https://www.drfuhrman.com:** A doctor's recommendation for nutritious recipes with video demonstrations.
- **https://www.doctorgaby.com:** Alan Gaby, MD, wrote the textbook *Nutritional Medicine*, which is Dana's bible.
- **http://www.greenmedinfo.com:** This site a great resource for learning about plant-based resources. It is the most widely

cited, open-access, evidence-based natural health resource, with more than twenty thousand articles.

- **https://www.greensmoothiegirl.com:** Robyn Openshaw has been an advocate for the health benefits of green smoothies for more than twenty years. Her website contains many green smoothie recipes.
- **https://www.heartmdinstitute.com:** Cardiologist Dr. Stephen Sinatra's website offers health and wellness information.
- **http://www.drhoffman.com:** Dr. Ronald Hoffman (Dana's mentor and friend) has a great podcast that gives great health advice.
- **https://www.lifespa.com:** Dr. John Douillard offers Ayurvedic advice and is also an expert on breathing, hydration, and high-performance athletics.
- **https://www.drmercola.com:** Widely read website providing free health and wellness articles.
- **https://www.t-tapp.com:** Teresa Tapp provides free resources and fifteen-minute full-body workouts that include fascia stretching.
- **https://www.thetappingsolution.com:** Nick Ortner brought global awareness to the stress-reduction technique called the Tapping Solution.

ENVIRONMENTAL WEBSITES, WATER CHARITIES, AND NONPROFITS

- **https://www.ewg.org:** This is the organization that listed the "dirty dozen" fruits and vegetables that should always be organic when possible and the "clean fifteen" that don't have to be organic. This site also has the following consumer resources:

Water filter buying guide
National tap water database
Shopper's guide to pesticides in produce
Guide to healthy cleaning
Guide to sunscreens
Consumer guide to seafood
Guide to safer cell phone use
Shopper's guide to avoiding GMO food

- **https://www.greenwave.org:** This site promotes ocean farming of seaweed and shellfish to mitigate climate change and provide kelp as a viable and superhealthy food source.
- **https://www.heifer.org:** This is a great charity that helps poverty and hunger by supplying farm animals to needy people so they can have sustainable food and reliable income.
- **http://www.rainforestflow.org:** This organization brings clean water to the indigenous peoples of the Amazon.
- **https://www.weareprojectzero.org:** Project Zero is dedicated to restoring and protecting our oceans.
- **http://www.container-recycling.org:** This organization provides research and education on ways to reduce waste, reuse, and recycling with an excellent database about these issues.
- **http://www.findaspring.com:** This site helps you locate natural springs around the world.
- **https://www.plasticoceans.org:** Get informed with this site that is dedicated to educating people on plastics and the oceans.

- **https://smile.amazon.com:** Let's face it: We all use Amazon, and this is a great way to give a portion to your charity of choice at no cost to you.
- **https://www.westonaprice.org:** The Weston A. Price Foundation is dedicated to restoring nutrient-dense foods to the human diet through education, research, and activism.

SOURCES FOR FINDING LIKE-MINDED DOCTORS

- **http://www.acam.org**
- **https://www.ifm.org**

RECOMMENDED SITES FOR MEDITATIVE PRACTICES

- **https://www.heartmath.com:** Inner balance is a great tool for breathing work that gives you instant biofeedback. Well studied and effective for anxiety, depression, and sleep disturbance.
- **https://www.rewireme.com:** This is a great informational website providing resources for mindfulness, spirituality, and neuroscience.
- **https://www.tm.org:** A great site for learning transcendental meditation.
- **https://www.instituteofintegralqigongandtaichi .org:** Provides information on meditation and movement.

Notes

INTRODUCTION: HYDRATION: HOW CAN WE DO IT BETTER?

1. Ericson, John. "75% of Americans May Suffer from Chronic Dehydration, According to Doctors." Medical Daily. Accessed June 25, 2017. http://www.medicaldaily.com/75-americans-may-suffer-chronic-dehydration-according-doctors-247393.
2. Thornton, Simon N., and Marie Trabalon. "Chronic Dehydration Is Associated with Obstructive Sleep Apnoea Syndrome." *Clinical Science* 128, no. 3 (February 1, 2015): 225. http://www.clinsci.org/content/128/3/225.
3. Chang, Tammy, et al. "Inadequate Hydration, BMI, and Obesity Among US Adults: NHANES 2009–2012." *Annals of Family Medicine* 14, no. 4 (July–August 2016): 320–324. Accessed October 22, 2017. http://www.annfammed.org/content/14/4/320.
4. Dennis, E. A., et al. "Water Consumption Increases Weight Loss During a Hypocaloric Diet Intervention in Middle-Aged and Older Adults." *Obesity* (Silver Spring) 18, no. 2 (February 2010): 300–307. Accessed October 22, 2017. https://www.ncbi.nlm.nih.gov/pubmed/19661958.
5. Preachuk, Deb. "The Connection Between Chronic Pain and Chronic Dehydration." Pain Free Posture MN. Accessed October 22, 2017. http://www.painfreeposturemn.com/the-connection-between-chronic-pain-and-chronic-dehydration.
6. Adan, A. "Cognitive Performance and Dehydration." *Journal of the American College of Nutrition* 31, no. 2 (April 2012): 71–78. Accessed October 25, 2017. https://www.ncbi.nlm.nih.gov/pubmed/?term=adan%2C%2Bcognitive%2Bperformance%2C%2B2012.

7. Bear, Tracey, et al. "A Preliminary Study on How Hypohydration Affects Pain Perception." *Psychophysiology* 53, no. 5 (May 2016): 605–610. Accessed October 22, 2017. https://www.ncbi.nlm.nih.gov/pubmed/26785699; doi:10.1111/psyp.12610.

   Moyen, N. E., et al. "Hydration Status Affects Mood State and Pain Sensation during Ultra-Endurance Cycling." *Journal of Sports Sciences* 33, no. 18 (March 2015): 1962–1969. Accessed October 22, 2017. https://www.ncbi.nlm.nih.gov/pubmed/25793570.

8. Armstrong, L. E., et al. "Mild Dehydration Affects Mood in Healthy Young Women." *Journal of Nutrition* 142, no. 2 (February 2012): 382–388. Accessed October 22, 2017. https://www.ncbi.nlm.nih.gov/pubmed/22190027.

9. Container Recycling Institute, http://www.container-recycling.org/index.php.

10. Langmead, L., R. J. Makins, and D. S. Rampton. "Anti-inflammatory Effects of Aloe Vera Gel in Human Colorectal Mucosa in Vitro." *Alimentary Pharmacology and Therapeutics* 19, no. 5 (March 1, 2004): 521–527. https://www.ncbi.nlm.nih.gov/pubmed/14987320; doi:10.1111/j.1365-2036.2004.01874.x.

CHAPTER 1: THE NEW SCIENCE OF WATER

1. Arnaoutis, Giannis, et al. "The Effect of Hypohydration on Endothelial Function in Young, Healthy Adults." *European Journal of Nutrition* 56, no. 3 (April 2017): 1211–1217. https://link.springer.com/article/10.1007%2Fs00394-016-1170-8.

2. Harvard Health Publishing, "Surprising Heart Attack and Stroke Triggers—from Waking up to Volcanoes." July 2007. https://www.health.harvard.edu/press_releases/heart-attack-triggers.

3. Mayo Clinic, Diabetic Ketoacidosis. http://www.mayoclinic.org/diseases-conditions/diabetic-ketoacidosis/basics/definition/con-20026470.

4. Manz, Friedrich, and Andreas Wentz. "The Importance of Good Hydration for the Prevention of Chronic Diseases." *Nutrition Reviews* 63, no 6 (2005). http://onlinelibrary.wiley.com/doi/10.1111/j.1753-4887.2005.tb00150.x/epdf.

5. Gonzalez, Nicholas. "Water, Energy, and the Perils of Dehydration." GreenMedInfo Blog. July 2, 2015. Accessed October 22, 2017. http://www.greenmedinfo.com/blog/water-energy-and-perils-dehydration.

6. Barnard College, Columbia University. The Facts About Laxatives. https://barnard.edu/counseling/resources/eating-disorders/laxatives.

7. Batmanghelidj, F. "A New and Natural Method of Treatment of Peptic Ulcer Disease." *Journal of Clinical Gastroenterology* 5, no. 3 (1983): 203–206.

8. Galson, Steven K. "Prevention of Deep Vein Thrombosis and Pulmonary Embolism." *Public Health Reports* 123, no. 4 (2008): 420–421. https://www.ncbi.nlm.nih.gov/pmc/articles/PMC2430635/; doi:10.1177/003335490812300402.

9. Ghosh, Arunava, R. C. Boucher, and Robert Tarran. "Airway Hydration and COPD." *Cellular and Molecular Life Sciences* 72, no. 19 (2015): 3637–3652. https://www.ncbi.nlm.nih.gov/pubmed/26068443; doi:10.1007/s00018-015-1946-7.

10. Gaby, A. R. "The Role of Hidden Food Allergy/Intolerance in Chronic Disease." *Alternative Medicine Review. A Journal of Clinical Therapeutics* 3, no. 2 (April 1998): 90–100. Accessed October 25, 2017. https://www.ncbi.nlm.nih.gov/pubmed/9577245.

11. Armstrong, L. E., et al. "Mild Dehydration Affects Mood in Healthy Young Women." *Journal of Nutrition* 142, no. 2 (February 2012): 382–388. Accessed October 25, 2017. https://www.ncbi.nlm.nih.gov/pubmed/22190027.

12. Benton, David. "Dehydration Influences Mood and Cognition: A Plausible Hypothesis?" *Nutrients* 3, no. 5 (May 2011): 555–573. https://www.ncbi.nlm.nih.gov/pmc/articles/PMC3257694/; doi:10.3390/nu3050555.

13. Thornton, Simon N. "Diabetes and Hypertension, as Well as Obesity and Alzheimer's Disease, Are Linked to Hypohydration-Induced Lower Brain Volume." *Frontiers in Aging Neuroscience* 6 (2014): 279. https://www.ncbi.nlm.nih.gov/pmc/articles/PMC4195368/; doi:10.3389/fnagi.2014.00279.

14. Ibid.

15. Dickson, J. M., et al. "The Effects of Dehydration on Brain Volume—Preliminary Results." *International Journal of Sports Medicine* 26, no. 6 (July–August 2005): 481–485. Accessed October 25, 2017. https://www.ncbi.nlm.nih.gov/pubmed/16037892.

16. Chumlea, W. C., et al. "Total Body Water Data for White Adults 18 to 64 Years of Age: The Fels Longitudinal Study." *Kidney International* 56, no. 1 (July 1999): 244–252. Accessed October 25, 2017. https://www.ncbi.nlm.nih.gov/pubmed/10411699.

17. Ritz, P., et al. "Influence of Gender and Body Composition on Hydration and Body Water Spaces." *Clinical Nutrition* 27, no. 5 (October 2008): 740–746. Accessed October 25, 2017. https://www.ncbi.nlm.nih.gov/pubmed/18774628.

18. Thornton, S. N. "Thirst and Hydration: Physiology and Consequences of Dysfunction." *Physiology and Behavior* 100, no. 1 (April 26, 2010): 15–21. Accessed October 26, 2017. https://www.ncbi.nlm.nih.gov/pubmed/20211637.

19. Beauchet, O., et al. "Blood Pressure Levels and Brain Volume Reduction: A Systematic Review and Meta-analysis." *Journal of Hypertension* 31, no. 8 (August 2013): 1502–1516. Accessed October 26, 2017. https://www.ncbi .nlm.nih.gov/pubmed/23811995.

20. Smith, David W., et al. "Altitude Modulates Concussion Incidence." *Orthopaedic Journal of Sports Medicine* 1, no. 6 (November 2013): 232596711351158. https://www.ncbi.nlm.nih.gov/pmc/articles/PMC4555510/; doi:10.1177/23 25967113511588.

21. Seneff, Stephanie, and Wendy A. Morley. "Diminished Brain Resilience Syndrome: A Modern Day Neurological Pathology of Increased Susceptibility to Mild Brain Trauma, Concussion, and Downstream Neurodegeneration." *Surgical Neurology International* 5, no. 1 (June 2014): 97. https://www .ncbi.nlm.nih.gov/pubmed/25024897; doi:10.4103/2152-7806.134731

22. University of North Carolina Chapel Hill, "NFL Grant Funds International Research on the Role of Active Rehabilitation Strategies in Concussion Management," news release, June 14, 2017. http://uncnews.unc .edu/2017/06/14/nfl-grant-funds-international-research-role-active -rehabilitation-strategies-concussion-management/.

23. "Concussion." Mayo Clinic. July 29, 2017. Accessed October 26, 2017. http://www.mayoclinic.org/diseases-conditions/concussion/symptoms -causes/dxc-20273155.

24. Seneff, Stephanie, and Wendy A. Morley. "Diminished Brain Resilience Syndrome: A Modern Day Neurological Pathology of Increased Susceptibility to Mild Brain Trauma, Concussion, and Downstream Neurodegeneration." *Surgical Neurology International* 5, no. 1 (June 2014): 97. https://www.ncbi .nlm.nih.gov/pubmed/25024897; doi:10.4103/2152-7806.134731.

25. "Concussion." Mayo Clinic. July 29, 2017. Accessed October 26, 2017. http://www.mayoclinic.org/diseases-conditions/concussion/symptoms -causes/dxc-20273155.

26. Bear, Tracey, et al. "A Preliminary Study on How Hypohydration Affects Pain Perception." *Psychophysiology* 53, no. 5 (May 2016): 605–610. https:// www.ncbi.nlm.nih.gov/pubmed/26785699; doi:10.1111/psyp.12610.

27. Ogino, Yuichi, et al. "Dehydration Enhances Pain-Evoked Activation in the Human Brain Compared with Rehydration." *Anesthesia and Analgesia* 118, no. 6 (June 2014): 1317–13325. https://www.ncbi.nlm.nih.gov/ pubmed/24384865; doi:10.1213/ane.0b013e3182a9b028.

28. "Lack of Sleep Is Affecting Americans, Finds the National Sleep Foundation." National Sleep Foundation. Accessed October 22, 2017. https://sleepfoundation.org/media-center/press-release/lack-sleep-affecting-americans-finds-the-national-sleep-foundation.

29. Xie, L., et al. "Sleep Drives Metabolite Clearance from the Adult Brain." *Science* 342, no. 6156 (October 18, 2013): 373–377. http://science.sciencemag.org/content/342/6156/373; doi:10.1126/science.1241224.

30. Jessen, Nadia Aalling, et al. "The Glymphatic System: A Beginner's Guide." *Neurochemical Research* 40, no. 12 (December 2015): 2583–2599. https://www.ncbi.nlm.nih.gov/pubmed/25947369; doi:10.1007/s11064-015-1581-6.

31. Mendelsohn, Andrew R., and James W. Larrick. "Sleep Facilitates Clearance of Metabolites from the Brain: Glymphatic Function in Aging and Neurodegenerative Diseases." *Rejuvenation Research* 16, no. 6 (December 2013): 518–523. https://www.ncbi.nlm.nih.gov/pubmed/24199995; doi:10.1089/rej.2013.1530.

32. Altieri, A., C. La Vecchia, and E. Negri. "Fluid Intake and Risk of Bladder and Other Cancers." *European Journal of Clinical Nutrition* 57 Supplement 2 (December 2003): S59–S68. https://www.ncbi.nlm.nih.gov/pubmed/14681715; doi:10.1038/sj.ejcn.1601903.

33. Vanderbilt University Medical Center. "Water's Unexpected Role in Blood Pressure Control." ScienceDaily. Accessed October 25, 2017. https://www.sciencedaily.com/releases/2010/07/100706150639.htm.

34. Boschmann, Michael, et al. "Water-Induced Thermogenesis." *Journal of Clinical Endocrinology and Metabolism* 88, no. 12 (December 2003): 6015–6019. https://www.ncbi.nlm.nih.gov/pubmed/14671205; doi:10.1210/jc.2003-030780.

35. Yang, Qing. "Gain Weight by 'Going Diet'? Artificial Sweeteners and the Neurobiology of Sugar Cravings." *Yale Journal of Biology and Medicine.* June 2010. Accessed October 25, 2017. https://www.ncbi.nlm.nih.gov/pmc/articles/PMC2892765/.

36. Howard, Jacqueline. "Diet Sodas May Be Tied to Stroke, Dementia Risk." CNN. April 20, 2017. Accessed October 25, 2017. http://www.cnn.com/2017/04/20/health/diet-sodas-stroke-dementia-study/index.html.

37. Bria, Rebecca. "Ritual, Economy, and the Production of Community at Ancient Hualcayan (Ancash, Peru)" (dissertation, Vanderbilt University, Department of Anthropology, 2017).

38. Perakis, Fivos, et al. "Diffusive Dynamics During the High-to-Low Density Transition in Amorphous Ice." *Proceedings of the National Academy of Sciences* 114, no. 31 (August 1, 2017): 8193–8198. http://www.pnas.org/content/114/31/8193; doi:10.1073/pnas.1705303114.

39. Crew, Bec. "Physicists Just Discovered a Second State of Liquid Water." ScienceAlert. November 14, 2016. Accessed October 23, 2017. https://www.sciencealert.com/physicists-just-discovered-a-second-state-of-liquid-water.

40. Saykally, R. J., and F. N. Keutsch. "Water Clusters: Untangling the Mysteries of the Liquid, One Molecule at a Time," *PNAS* 98, no. 19 (September 2001): 10533–10540.

41. McGeoch, Julie E. M., and Malcolm W. McGeoch. "Entrapment of Water by Subunit C of ATP Synthase." *Journal of the Royal Society Interface* 5, no. 20 (March 6, 2008): 311–318. Accessed October 23, 2017. http://rsif.royalsociety publishing.org/content/5/20/311.

42. Kang, Young-Rye, et al. "Anti-obesity and Anti-diabetic Effects of Yerba Mate (*Ilex Paraguariensis*) in C57BL/6J Mice Fed a High-Fat Diet." *Laboratory Animal Research* 28, no. 1 (March 2012): 23–29. Accessed October 23, 2017. https://www.ncbi.nlm.nih.gov/pmc/articles/PMC3315195/.

43. Pollack, Gerald. "The Fourth Phase of Water." The Weston A. Price Foundation. February 15, 2016. Accessed October 23, 2017. https://www.westona price.org/health-topics/health-issues/the-fourth-phase-of-water/.

44. Xu, Chen, et al. "Light-Harvesting Chlorophyll Pigments Enable Mammalian Mitochondria to Capture Photonic Energy and Produce ATP." *Journal of Cell Science* (January 15, 2014). Accessed October 23, 2017. http://jcs.biologists.org/content/127/2/388.

CHAPTER 2: EAT YOUR WATER

1. Valtin, Heinz, with the technical assistance of Sheila A. Gorman. "'Drink at Least Eight Glasses of Water a Day.' Really? Is There Scientific Evidence for '8 × 8'?" *American Journal of Physiology—Regulatory, Integrative and Comparative Physiology* 283, no. 5 (November 1, 2002): R993–R1004. Accessed October 25, 2017. http://ajpregu.physiology.org/content/283/5/R993. *See also* Carroll, Aaron E. "No, You Do Not Have to Drink 8 Glasses of Water a Day." *New York Times*, August 24, 2015.

2. "How Much Feed and Water Are Used to Make a Pound of Beef?" Beef Cattle Research Council. Accessed October 25, 2017. http://www.beef research.ca/blog/cattle-feed-water-use/.

3. Ibrahim, Fandi, et al. "Probiotic Bacteria as Potential Detoxification Tools: Assessing Their Heavy Metal Binding Isotherms." *Canadian Journal*

of Microbiology 52, no. 9 (September 2006): 877–885. https://www.ncbi .nlm.nih.gov/pubmed/17110980; doi 10.1139/w06-043.

4. Gordon, J. I, and J. Xu. "Honor Thy Symbionts." *Proceedings of the National Academy of Sciences* 100, no. 18 (September 2, 2003): 10452–10459. http:// www.pnas.org/content/100/18/10452.abstract.

5. Smits, Samuel A., et al. "Seasonal Cycling in the Gut Microbiome of the Hadza Hunter-Gatherers of Tanzania." *Science* 357, no. 6353 (August 25, 2017): 802–806. Accessed October 25, 2017. http://science.sciencemag .org/content/357/6353/802.

6. Pall, Martin L. "Microwave Frequency Electromagnetic Fields (EMFs) Produce Widespread Neuropsychiatric Effects Including Depression." *Journal of Chemical Neuroanatomy* 75 Part 3 (September 2016): 43–51. https:// www.ncbi.nlm.nih.gov/pubmed/26300312; doi:10.1016/j.jchemneu.2015 .08.001.

7. Spector, Tim, and Jeff Leach. "I Spent Three Days as a Hunter-Gatherer to See If It Would Improve My Gut Health." The Conversation. June 30, 2017. Accessed October 25, 2017. http://theconversation.com/i-spent-three-days-as -a-hunter-gatherer-to-see-if-it-would-improve-my-gut-health-78773.

8. Smits et al. "Seasonal Cycling in the Gut Microbiome of the Hadza Hunter-Gatherers of Tanzania." *Science* 357, no. 6353 (August 25, 2017): 802–806. Accessed October 25, 2017. http://science.sciencemag.org/content/357/ 6353/802.

CHAPTER 3: MOVE THAT WATER

1. Oschman, J. L. *Energy Medicine in Therapeutics and Human Performance.*, London: Elsevier, 2003.

2. *Strolling Under the Skin: Images of Living Matter Architectures*, directed by Jean-Claude Guimberteau (2005), DVD. www.endovivo.com.

3. Views of the Living Fascia: https://www.youtube.com/watch?v=qSXpX4 wyoY8.

4. Pienta, K. J., and D. S. Coffey. "Cellular Harmonic Information Transfer Through a Tissue Tensegrity-Matriux System," *Medical Hypotheses* 34 (1991): 88–95.

5. Ho, M. W. "First Sighting of Structured Water," *Science in Society* 28 (2005): 47–48; *See also* Ho, M. W. "Positive Electricity Zaps Through Water Chains," *Science in Society* 28 (2005): 49–50; Ho, M. W. "Collagen

Water Structure Revealed," *Science in Society* 32 (2006): 15–16; Ho, M. W. *Living Rainbow H₂O,* London: World Scientific and Imperial College Press, 2012; Ho, M. W. "Living H₂O," *Science in Society* 55 (2017).

6. Ji, Sungchul. *The Cell Language Theory.* London: World Scientific Publishing Company, 2017.

7. For a detailed discussion of Fuller's thinking, go to Dr. Stephen M. Levin's website, http://www.biotensegrity.com.

8. Myers, Thomas. *Fascial Release for Structural Balance.* Berkeley, CA: North Atlantic Books, 2010, 2017.

9. Schleip, Robert, "Fascia as a Sensory Organ" (webinar, World Massage Conference Webinar, 2009).

10. Langevin, H. M., et al. "Evidence of Connective Tissue Involvement in Acupuncture," *FASEB Journal* express article 10.1096/fj.01-0925fje. Published online April 10, 2002.

CHAPTER 4: HOW MOTION KEEPS YOU HYDRATED

1. Hagger-Johnson, G., et al. "Sitting Time, Fidgeting and All-Cause Mortality in the UK Women's Cohort Study." *American Journal of Preventive Medicine* 50, no. 2 (2016): 154–160.

2. Morishima, Takuma, et al. "Prolonged Sitting-Induced Leg Endothelial Dysfunction Is Prevented by Fidgeting." *American Journal of Physiology Heart and Circulatory Physiology* 311, no. 1 (July 1, 2016): H177–H182. Published online May 27, 2016.

3. Bagriantsev, Sviatoslav N., Elena O. Gracheva, and Patrick G. Gallagher. "Piezo Proteins: Regulators of Mechanosensation and Other Cellular Processes." *Journal of Biological Chemistry* 289 (November 14, 2014): 31673–31681. Accessed October 25, 2017. http://www.jbc.org/content/289/46/31673.full.

4. Doidge, Norman. *The Brain That Changes Itself: Stories of Personal Triumph from the Frontiers of Brain Science.* New York: Viking, 2007.

5. Ortner, Nick. *The Tapping Solution for Pain Relief: A Step-by-Step Guide to Reducing and Eliminating Chronic Pain.* Carlsbad, CA: Hay House, 2015.

6. Feinstein, David. "Acupoint Stimulation in Treating Psychological Disorders: Evidence of Efficacy." *Review of General Psychology* 16, no. 4 (2012): 364–380. https://www.researchgate.net/publication/263918679_Acupoint_Stimulation_in_Treating_Psychological_Disorders_Evidence_of_Efficacy; doi:10.1037/a0028602.

CHAPTER 5: FAT AND HYDRATION

1. Cao, Jing, et al. "Incorporation and Clearance of Omega-3 Fatty Acids in Erythrocyte Membranes and Plasma Phospholipids." *Clinical Chemistry* 52, no. 12 (December 2006): 2262–2272. Accessed October 25, 2017. https://experts.umn.edu/en/publications/incorporation-and-clearance-of-omega-3-fatty-acids-in-erythrocyte.

2. Darios, Frédéric, and Bazbek Davletov. "Omega-3 and Omega-6 Fatty Acids Stimulate Cell Membrane Expansion by Acting on Syntaxin||3." *Nature* 440 (April 6, 2006): 813–817. Accessed October 25, 2017. https://www.nature.com/nature/journal/v440/n7085/abs/nature04598.html.

3. Bazan, N. G., A. E. Musto, and E. J. Knott. "Endogenous Signaling by Omega-3 Docosahexaenoic Acid-Derived Mediators Sustains Homeostatic Synaptic and Circuitry Integrity." *Molecular Neurobiology* 44, no. 2 (October 2011): 216–222. Accessed October 25, 2017. https://www.ncbi.nlm.nih.gov/pubmed/21918832.

4. http://www.ific.org/research/foodandhealthsurvey.cfm and via authors' interview with Shelley Goldberg, MPH, RD, senior director of nutrition communications for the International Food Information Council.

5. Roberts M. N., et al. "A Ketogenic Diet Extends Longevity and Healthspan in Adult Mice." *Cell Metabolism* 26, no. 3 (2017): 539–546. http://www.cell.com/cell-metabolism/fulltext/S1550-4131(17)30490-4.

6. Jiang, Yan, and Wen-Jing Nie. "Chemical Properties in Fruits of Mulberry Species from the Xinjiang Province of China." *Food Chemistry* 174 (May 1, 2015): 460–466. Accessed October 25, 2017. http://www.sciencedirect.com/science/article/pii/S0308814614018123.

7. Howard B. V., et al. "Low-Fat Dietary Pattern and Risk of Cardiovascular Disease: The Women's Health Initiative Randomized Controlled Dietary Modification Trial." *Journal of the American Medical Association* 295, no. 6 (February 8, 2006): 655–666. https://www.ncbi.nlm.nih.gov/pubmed/16467234; doi:10.1001/jama.295.6.655.

8. Dehghan, Mahshid, et al. "Associations of Fats and Carbohydrate Intake with Cardiovascular Disease and Mortality in 18 Countries from Five Continents (PURE): A Prospective Cohort Study." *Lancet* 390, no. 10107 (November 4–10, 2017): 2050–2062. Accessed October 26, 2017. https://www.sciencedirect.com/science/article/pii/S0140673617322523.

9. Brown, Elizabeth Nolan. "More Evidence That Everything the Government Teaches Us About Eating Is Wrong." *Hit & Run* (blog). Reason

.com. August 30, 2017. Accessed October 25, 2017. http://reason.com/blog/2017/08/30/pure-study-challenges-dietary-dogma.

10. Unlu, Nuray Z., et al. "Carotenoid Absorption from Salad and Salsa by Humans Is Enhanced by the Addition of Avocado or Avocado Oil." *Journal of Nutrition* 135, no. 3 (March 1, 2005): 431–436. Accessed October 25, 2017. http://jn.nutrition.org/cgi/content/full/135/3/431.

11. Gardner, Christopher D., et al. "Comparison of the Atkins, Zone, Ornish, and LEARN Diets for Change in Weight and Related Risk Factors Among Overweight Premenopausal Women." *Journal of the American Medical Association* 297, no. 9 (March 7, 2007): 969–977. https://www.ncbi.nlm.nih.gov/pubmed/17341711; doi:10.1001/jama.297.9.969.

12. Mylonas, C., and D. Kouretas. "Lipid Peroxidation and Tissue Damage." *In Vivo* 13, no. 3 (May–June 1999): 295–309. Accessed October 26, 2017. https://www.ncbi.nlm.nih.gov/pubmed/10459507.

CHAPTER 6: WHO NEEDS WATER THE MOST?

1. Report on the Hydration Pilot Project at the Ideal School. Hydration Foundation. https://www.hydrationfoundation.org.

2. Kenney, E. L., et al. "Prevalence of Inadequate Hydration Among US Children and Disparities by Gender and Race/Ethnicity: National Health and Nutrition Examination Survey, 2009–2012." *American Journal of Public Health* 105, no. 8 (August 2015): e113–e118. Accessed October 25, 2017. https://www.ncbi.nlm.nih.gov/pubmed/26066941.

3. Wang, ZiMian, et al. "Specific Metabolic Rates of Major Organs and Tissues Across Adulthood: Evaluation by Mechanistic Model of Resting Energy Expenditure." *American Journal of Clinical Nutrition* 92, no. 6 (December 2010): 1369–1377. Accessed October 25, 2017. https://www.ncbi.nlm.nih.gov/pmc/articles/PMC2980962/.

4. State Government of Victoria, Australia. Department of Health and Human Services. "Sweat." Better Health Channel. August 31, 2015. Accessed October 25, 2017. https://www.betterhealth.vic.gov.au/health/conditionsandtreatments/sweat.

5. "The Smell Report: Sexual Attraction." Social Issues Research Centre. Accessed October 25, 2017. http://www.sirc.org/publik/smell_attract.html.

6. "What's Sweat?" KidsHealth. Nemours Foundation. Accessed October 25, 2017. http://m.kidshealth.org/en/kids/sweat.html.

7. Murray, Bob. "Hydration and Physical Performance." *Journal of the American College of Nutrition* 26, sup. 5 (2007): 542S–548S. Taylor and Francis Online. Accessed October 26, 2017. http://www.tandfonline.com/doi/full/10.1080/07315724.2007.10719656.

8. American College of Sports Medicine, "Selecting and Effectively Using Hydration for Fitness," 2011. www.acsm.org/docs/brochures/selecting-and-effectively-using-hydration-for-fitness.pdf.

9. "Hyponatremia." Mayo Clinic. May 28, 2014. Accessed October 25, 2017. http://www.mayoclinic.org/diseases-conditions/hyponatremia/basics/definition/con-20031445.

10. "Hyponatremia in Athletes." Gatorade Sports Science Institute. Accessed October 26, 2017. http://www.gssiweb.org/en/sports-science-exchange/article/sse-88-hyponatremia-in-athletes.

11. Lewis, M. D., and J. Bailes. "Neuroprotection for the Warrior: Dietary Supplementation with Omega-3 Fatty Acids." *Military Medicine* 176, no. 10 (October 2011): 1120–1127. Accessed October 26, 2017. https://www.ncbi.nlm.nih.gov/pubmed/22128646.

12. Popkin, Barry M., Kristen E. D'Anci, and Irwin H. Rosenberg. "Water, Hydration, and Health." *Nutrition Reviews* 68, no. 8 (August 2010): 439–458. Accessed October 25, 2017. http://onlinelibrary.wiley.com/doi/10.1111/j.1753-4887.2010.00304.x/abstract.

13. Hooper, L., S. Whitelock, and D. Bunn. "Reducing Dehydration in Residents of Care Homes." *Nursing Times* 111, nos. 34–35 (August 19–September 1, 2015): 16–19. Accessed October 25, 2017. https://www.ncbi.nlm.nih.gov/pubmed/26492664.

14. Boskabady, M. H., et al. "Pharmacological Effects of *Rosa Damascena*." *Iranian Journal of Basic Medical Sciences* 14, no. 4 (July–August 2011): 295–307. Accessed October 26, 2017. https://www.ncbi.nlm.nih.gov/pmc/articles/PMC3586833/; http://europepmc.org/articles/PMC3586833.

15. Hooper, L., S. Whitelock, and D. Bunn. "Reducing Dehydration in Residents of Care Homes." *Nursing Times* 111, nos. 34–35 (August 19–September 1, 2015): 16–19. Accessed October 25, 2017. https://www.ncbi.nlm.nih.gov/pubmed/26492664.

CHAPTER 7: ANTIAGING, THE SKIN, AND BEAUTY

1. Genuis, S., et al. "Human Elimination of Phthalate Compounds: Blood, Urine, and Sweat (BUS) Study." *Scientific World Journal* (2012): 615068.

2. Patrick, Rhonda. *Hyperthermic Conditioning's Role in Increasing Endurance, Muscle Mass, and Neurogenesis.* Report. 2017. https://www.foundmyfitness.com.

3. Wunsch, Alexander, and Karsten Matuschka. "A Controlled Trial to Determine the Efficacy of Red and Near-Infrared Light Treatment in Patient Satisfaction, Reduction of Fine Lines, Wrinkles, Skin Roughness, and Intradermal Collagen Density Increase." *Photomedicine and Laser Surgery* 32, no. 2 (February 1, 2014): 93–100. Government of Canada. National Research Council Canada. Accessed October 25, 2017. http://pubmedcentralcanada.ca/pmcc/articles/PMC3926176/.

4. Xie, Lulu, et al. "Sleep Drives Metabolite Clearance from the Adult Brain." *Science* 342, no. 6156 (October 18, 2013): 373–377. Accessed October 25, 2017. http://science.sciencemag.org/content/342/6156/373.

5. Kapandji, I. A. *The Physiology of the Joints: Annotated Diagrams of the Mechanics of the Human Joints.* Vol. 1. Edinburgh: Churchill Livingstone, 2007.

6. Amy Cuddy's TED Talk, "Your Body Language May Shape Who You Are." https://www.ted.com/talks/amy_cuddy_your_body_language_shapes_who_you_are/transcript.

7. Aslam, Muhammad Nadeem, Ephraim Philip Lansky, and James Varani. "Pomegranate as a Cosmeceutical Source: Pomegranate Fractions Promote Proliferation and Procollagen Synthesis and Inhibit Matrix Metalloproteinase-1 Production in Human Skin Cells." *Journal of Ethnopharmacology* 103, no. 3 (February 20, 2006): 311–318. University of Michigan. Michigan Experts. Accessed October 25, 2017. https://experts.umich.edu/en/publications/pomegranate-as-a-cosmeceutical-source-pomegranate-fractions-promo.

CHAPTER 8: THE QUENCH PLAN

1. Hooper, Lee, et al. "Water-Loss Dehydration and Aging." *Mechanisms of Ageing and Development* 136–137 (March–April 2014): 50–58. Accessed October 25, 2017. https://www.sciencedirect.com/science/article/pii/S0047637413001280. *See also* Hooper, L., S. Whitelock, and D. Bunn. "Reducing Dehydration in Residents of Care Homes." *Nursing Times* 111, nos. 34–35 (August 19–September 1, 2015): 16–19. Accessed October 25, 2017. https://www.ncbi.nlm.nih.gov/pubmed/26492664.

CHAPTER 9: THE CUP RUNNETH OVER

1. Toth, P. P. et al. "Bergamot Reduces Plasma Lipids, Atherogenic Small Dense LDL, and Subclinical Atherosclerosis in Subjects with Moderate Hypercholesterolemia: A 6 Months Prospective Study." *Frontiers in Pharmacology* 6 (January 6, 2016): 299. Accessed October 25, 2017. https://www.ncbi.nlm.nih.gov/pubmed/26779019.
2. Steinberg, F. M., M. M. Bearden, and C. L. Keen. "Cocoa and Chocolate Flavonoids: Implications for Cardiovascular Health." *Journal of the American Dietetic Association* 103, no. 2 (February 2003): 215–223. Accessed October 25, 2017. https://www.ncbi.nlm.nih.gov/pubmed/12589329.

APPENDIX

1. Crook, William G., and Cynthia P. Crook. *Tracking Down Hidden Food Allergy.* Jackson, TN: Professional Books, 1980.

Index

About the Authors

Dana G. Cohen, MD has been practicing integrative medicine for the last twenty years. She is currently the Medical Director of Complete Wellness, an integrated medical/wellness facility in the heart of Manhattan. She is on the scientific advisory board of the Organic & Natural Health Association and is an advisor to the board of directors for the American College for the Advancement in Medicine. As a world traveler, she loves to collect knowledge and stories of ancient and other cultures' healing practices. She lives in New York City.

Gina Bria, named Real World Scholar, is an anthropologist, author, and speaker who works on the forefront of water science and hydration. Head of the Hydration Foundation, she collects stories and strategies from cultures around the globe on how people find and use water. She speaks on the pressing need for hydration in our modern environments and her TEDx Talk "How to Grow Water: It's Not Only Blue, It's Green" provides surprising solutions for our water-challenged world. She consults and develops water projects around the globe and is a founding member of the World Wide Water and Health Association, a Senior Advisor to TEDx New York Salon, and a former Fellow with the Social Science Research Council. She lives in New York City.

For more information about the authors, visit www.drdana cohen.com and www.hydrationfoundation.org.